# Do You Use Food To Cope?

*ALSO BY DR. FORMAN*
SELF-FULLNESS: The Art of Loving and Caring for Your "Self"

# Do You Use Food To Cope?

## A Comprehensive 15-Week Program for Overcoming Emotional Overeating

*Sheila H. Forman, Ph.D.*

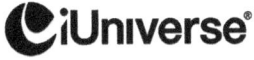

Do You Use Food To Cope?
A Comprehensive 15-Week Program for
Overcoming Emotional Overeating

Writers Club Press
an imprint of iUniverse, Inc.

iUniverse books may be ordered through booksellers or by contacting:

iUniverse
1663 Liberty Drive
Bloomington, IN 47403
www.iuniverse.com
1-800-Authors (1-800-288-4677)

ISBN: 978-0-5952-1280-4 (sc)

Print information available on the last page.

iUniverse rev. date: 04/10/2015

# DEDICATION

This book is dedicated to my parents Harry and Charlotte Forman for their unwavering faith in me. Thank you.

# DISCLAIMER

This book is designed to provide information in regard to the subject matter covered. It is sold with the understanding that the author is not engaged in rendering medical, psychological, psychiatric, or other professional advice or services.

If you have any physical or psychological condition that could be adversely affected, you are encouraged to seek the advice of an appropriate medical or mental health professional before beginning or continuing any of the suggestions made in this book.

The purpose of this book is to educate and encourage. The author shall have neither liability nor responsibility to any person or entity with respect to any loss or damage caused, or alleged to be caused, directly or indirectly, by the information contained in this book.

References made to patients are not references to specific people. Rather they are composites of many people put together for the purposes of illustration and instruction. Any resemblance to real persons, dead or alive, is purely coincidental.

ALL STRUGGLES HAVE A BEGINNING,
AN END, AND A PURPOSE.

# CONTENTS

Disclaimer ................................................................................vii

Acknowledgments ...................................................................xv

Why I Wrote This Book ..........................................................xvii

How To Use This Book ............................................................xix

Introduction .............................................................................xxi

Part One: Understanding Emotional Overeating ........................1

    *What is Emotional Eating?* ....................................................*4*

    *Understanding Anorexia and Bulimia* ..................................*5*

    *What is Anorexia Nervosa?* ...................................................*5*

    *What is Bulimia Nervosa?* .....................................................*6*

    *What is Binge Eating Disorder?* .............................................*7*

    *How Do You Know If You Have an Eating Disorder?* .............*8*

    *Treating Eating Disorders* ......................................................*8*

    *Why Do You Overeat?* ...........................................................*9*

    *What Kind of Overeater Are You?* ........................................*11*

    *How People Become Overeaters* .............................................*13*

    *Dieting or Restrictive Eating* ...............................................*16*

    *Food Triggers* .......................................................................*16*

    *It is Also About Self-Esteem* ................................................*17*

    *Eating and Weight are Just Symptoms* .................................*19*

    *Why People Gain Weight* ......................................................*20*

    *Overeating is Learned Behavior* ...........................................*24*

    *Overeating as Coping* ...........................................................*25*

Part Two: 15-Weeks To Overcoming Emotional Overeating ...........29

    *Week One: Acknowledging That You Are An Emotional Eater* ................*33*

*Week Two: Assessing Your Readiness*
   *To Change The Way You Live Your Life* ...............38
*Week Three: Your Diet And Weight History* ............45
*Week Four: Admitting That Diets Don't Work* ...........49
*Week Five: Accepting Your Body And Your Weight For Now* ..........56
*Week Six: Getting Rid Of The Scale* .................60
*Week Seven: Making Food Conscious –*
   *Using Your Food Awareness Inventory* ...........66
*Week Eight: Relating To Your Emotions –*
   *Using Your Emotion Awareness Inventory* ............69
*Week Nine: Discovering Your True Hungers –*
   *Recognizing WHEN You Overeat* ...........76
*Week Ten: Discovering Your True Hungers –*
   *Recognizing WHERE You Overeat* ............81
*Week Eleven: Discovering Your True Hungers*
   *Recognizing What Foods You Overeat* ...........85
*Week Twelve: Discovering Your True Hungers –*
   *Recognizing WHY You Overeat* ............88
*Week Thirteen: Learning New Ways To Cope* ..........106
*Week Fourteen: Relapse Prevention* ................118
*Week Fifteen: Putting It All Together Forever* ...........121

Part Three: When It Is Time To See A Professional ..........127
 *Getting Medical Attention* ...................129
 *Getting Psychological Attention* ................129
 *Choosing a Therapist* ....................131
 *Finding a Support Group* ..................132
 *Resources for Getting Help* ..................133
 *Treatment Facilities* .....................135

Part Four: The *Do You Use Food to Cope* Workbook ..........139
 *Food Awareness Inventory* ..................141

*Emotions Awareness Inventory* ............................................................ *151*
*My Hunger Inventory* ...................................................................... *160*
*My Recovery Diary* ......................................................................... *167*
*Plan of Action Worksheet* ............................................................... *184*
*My "Other Things To Do Instead of Eating" List* ............................. *185*
*Anger Letter* ................................................................................... *186*
*Love Myself Letter* ......................................................................... *187*
*My Journal* .................................................................................... *188*
*Rewards and Reinforcements* ........................................................... *193*
   *My Rewards and Reinforcements* .................................................. *193*
   *Rewards Chart* ......................................................................... *194*
   *Financial Rewards Chart* ........................................................... *195*
*Goal Setting Worksheet* ................................................................... *195*
*Forming Your Own Support Group* ................................................... *198*
*Photojournalism:* ............................................................................ *198*
*Other Strategies* .............................................................................. *201*

About The Author ......................................................................203

# ACKNOWLEDGMENTS

Writing the acknowledgments for my first book, *Self-fullness: The Art of Loving and Caring for Your 'Self'* was easy. The list was short and self evident. Writing the acknowledgments for this book is a much tougher task, mostly because so many people rallied around me after the publication of my first book and encouraged me to write this one that I don't know with whom to begin.

I suppose I will start with the three people whose caring, friendship, willingness, and expertise in "computerese" have brought my books to life. They are Robert A. Katz, Roger Barrett James, Esq., and David A. Smith. Without their help my ideas would be mere words on a page. Gentlemen, I thank you.

I also want to thank Professor Deborah Forman who lent me her spare laptop computer after I sent out a mass email looking for one to "buy, borrow, or steal!" Thank you Deb.

Thank you, too, to all the rest of you who responded to my email with your wonderful ideas, suggestions and solutions. Especially, Melanie Dreyfus, David Forman, Janene Forman, Lisa Khandelwal, Marilyn Jacobowitz, Tina Morgan, Tomas and Rachel Montoya, Steve Rosenberg, and Bruce Spiegel.

A huge thank you also goes out to Madge Beletsky, Jadranka Hyatt, Deirdre O'Connor, Debbie Goodman, Renee Gordon, Jack Nelson Soll, Laura Arnold, Maureen Friend, Elana Dixon, Beth Forman, Jim Hissong, Suzy Schultz, Nancy Jacobson, Bonnie Flink, Marji Pearson,

Linda Schutzer, Nancy Steiner, Roberta Kaye Friedman, and Ada Blumstein. You are all dear to me and I thank you for your support.

# WHY I WROTE THIS BOOK

For years, I have been a clinical psychologist working with women and men who struggle with food issues. Many of them overeat in response to stress and anxiety. Others overeat in response to joyful occasions or use food as a reward. Still others overeat in reaction to their latest dieting effort. During our work, I often want to recommend reading material to my patients to speed along their process of overcoming overeating and getting on with their lives. While there are many excellent books available, I found none that gives all the information I would like my patients to have.

This book contains, in my opinion, the basic material for anyone to start understanding their relationship with food and to learn how to get out of their emotional overeating dilemma and START LIVING! It also offers hope to those who have struggled for years with the "uncontrollable urge" to overeat in response to stress, anxiety, or any other uncomfortable emotion.

Included are many exercises and techniques that I have used successfully over the years with my patients. They are finally in one place and in a format that allows you to return to them as you make your journey from an emotional overeater to someone at peace with food.

I designed these exercises and techniques into a 15-week program that you can follow on your own or use with the help of a trained professional. In the sections that follow I offer some suggestion on how you can get the most out of the ideas and program described in this book.

[A note about gender. For ease of reading, I refer to the female gender throughout the book. This is not intended to suggest that only women suffer from emotional overeating. This book is of equal value to men who struggle with this issue. I hope my male readers do not take offense!]

# How To Use This Book

*Do You Use Food To Cope?* is divided into four parts. Part One offers some background information on emotional overeating and distinguishes it from a diagnosable eating disorder. If you have any suspicion that you may suffer from an eating disorder, such as Anorexia Nervosa or Bulimia Nervosa, I recommend that you begin with Part One. It may be necessary for you to consult with a physician or mental health professional before beginning your 15-week program.

Part Two is your 15-week program. While the program is divided into 15 weekly sessions, feel free to take more time to complete and adopt the information in each session. I do not recommend taking less than one week per session because it takes at least that long to grasp and internalize the concepts and ideas presented.

In Part Three you will find information on how to get professional assistance with this program or any aspect of it. I offer you names and telephone numbers of associations and organizations that can be of help.

Part Four is your *Do You Use Food To Cope?* Workbook. The tools you will use in the program plus much more are included in this part. You are welcome to write directly in the workbook or create your own using a journal or notebook of your choice.

I strongly recommend that you start with Part One to get a good understanding of what emotional eating is all about before you begin your 15-week program. For those of you who cannot wait another moment before tackling this problem, go directly to Part Two to begin. At some point, I hope you will choose to read Part One as well.

However you decide to use this book, I wish you much success at resolving once and for all your emotional relationship with food.

# INTRODUCTION

You feel you can't help it. You don't want to go to the refrigerator. You don't want to eat. You know you are not hungry and yet you can't seem to stop yourself. It's as if a magnetic force is pulling you into the kitchen, towards the food. You feel you have no control. You cannot stop this pull. You want to, but you can't. You feel helpless. You eat. You eat more. You tell yourself you are weak and bad and stupid. You hate yourself. You eat more. You are starting to feel full. You continue to eat. You want to stop. You can't stop. Now, you are starting to feel sick. Still you can't stop. You are getting tired. You are also getting tired of eating. You are starting to slow down. Finally you stop. You walk over to the couch or the table or the bed. You sit down. You hate yourself. You hate your life. You want to die.

This is the world of a binge. A horrible, self-destructive episode that knows no limits. The person who binges hates herself, hates her life, and hates her world. Fortunately, there *are* limits to a binge. Binge eating can be stopped. This book will show you how.

After many years of research and working with women and men who binge eat, I have learned the steps to overcoming overeating. They are simple steps but not necessarily easy ones. Come with me on this journey to peace with food. Over the next 15 weeks let me show you how to stop using food to feel better, how to cope with the stress and anxiety in your life without overeating, and how to break the chain between the urge to binge and the act of binge eating.

Before we begin, I want to tip my hat to you and offer you my sincerest congratulations for your decision to read this book. I know that the idea of finally being able to let go of bingeing is exhilarating. I also know that it can be very scary. I am pretty sure that this is not the first book you've read on the subject, nor is it your first attempt to stop overeating. You are probably a mixture of excitement and nervousness right now. That's okay. It is understandable. As you go along you may find yourself feeling anxious or uncomfortable. That's normal. It is expected. At times, you may start overeating more than before and certainly more than you want to now. That is also normal. It is a typical response to the emotions you will experience as you move through the program. Realize that if you have always used food to cope with your emotions, you will do so now too, for a time, until you learn the skills this book has to offer. Nowhere in this book will you ever read that it's not okay to eat. No where in this book will I ever tell you what to eat or how much. And most important nowhere in this book will I tell you to stop eating. You need to eat. I don't just mean for nutritional reasons. You need to eat for emotional reasons as well. Until you have the tools to deal with your life without overeating asking you to give up food as a coping mechanism would be detrimental. Eating serves a very important and valuable purpose for you. It is how you have managed to stay alive in your world. It is how you cope. It is what you do in response to the emotions you experience in your life. To take away your coping mechanism without giving you new ones in its place would create too much anxiety and send you head first into an enormous binge. I won't do that. You won't do that.

As you progress through this book you will learn why you overeat, what purpose it serves you and how you can stop. Go at your own pace. There is no such thing as failure. If you have a set back don't fret. It is part of the learning experience. You are about to embark on a lifetime journey of self-discovery and growth. This is the beginning of a healthy life filled with success and joy. So, grab your pen, highlighter or maker and let's get started!

# PART ONE:

## UNDERSTANDING EMOTIONAL OVEREATING

I want to begin by telling you the difference between an eating disorder, such as Anorexia Nervosa or Bulimia Nervosa, that requires professional attention and inappropriate emotional overeating which you can usually address on your own. Eating disorders are serious emotional and physical problems that can have life threatening consequences. They often arise from a combination of long standing psychological, emotional, and social experiences. Feelings of anxiety, depression, low self esteem, loneliness, as well as, interpersonal difficulties with families and friends may also contribute to the development of an eating disorder. Our society, with its emphasis on thinness and an unrealistic view of the "ideal" body may also play a role. Some people use dieting, bingeing, purging, and over exercising to cope with the pain in their life. Sometimes these behaviors help people feel in control of their situation. Once started these behavior can become habitual and undermine the person's emotional and physical well being.

The distinction between emotional overeating and having an eating disorder is very important. Many people walk around with the feeling that they have an eating disorder. They label themselves as "bulimic" or as a "compulsive overeater" and in so doing make it more difficult for them to stop the behavior. The label makes them feel their situation is hopeless. I want to assure you that even an "officially" diagnosed eating disordered person is not hopeless. Eating disorders, whether Anorexia Nervosa or Bulimia Nervosa, are currently being treated successfully by medical and mental health professionals all over the world. If you believe you may have anorexia or bulimia, I will make special recommendations for you as we go along.

**What is Emotional Eating?**
You are eating emotionally when you eat for reasons other than physical hunger. When you eat because you are anxious, you are emotionally eating. When you eat because you are happy, you are emotionally eating. Anytime you eat when you are not physically hungry you are eating for other reasons and those reasons as we shall see are usually emotional. Emotional eating tends to be episodic. It is often done secretively and usually involves high-calorie, high fat foods. Emotional overeating is not a diagnosable eating disorder.

Let me give you an example to help you better understand emotional eating. Lois is a 57 year old homemaker and mother of two grown daughters. She has been married for almost forty years and is considerably overweight. Lois has tried numerous diets and none has helped her weight problem. She says this is because every afternoon she sits in front of her television eating. She eats until she hears her husband come home. She quickly puts away her food and greets him at the door. Then she eats again with him when she serves dinner. She eats dinner even though she is not physically hungry because she doesn't want her husband to know that she spent the afternoon snacking. Lois' afternoon eating episodes contribute significantly to her weight problem. When I probed Lois about her afternoon binges she confessed that ever since her youngest daughter left home she has felt very lonely and empty. She is using the food (and the television) to fill up the loneliness in her life. This is classic emotional eating. What I helped Lois do is fill up her afternoon with other activities and people. With a little bit of coaxing I persuaded Lois to enroll in college and finish the degree she started so many years ago. By being busy with school, Lois no longer fills up her afternoons with food and is slowly losing the excess weight she carries.

**Understanding Anorexia and Bulimia**

To determine whether you have a diagnosable eating disorder ask yourself the following questions:

Do you:

- Often think about your body shape and weight?
- Feel fat, even though others say you are not?
- Consume large amounts of food in short periods of time?
- Fast, vomit, use laxatives or exercise a lot?
- Fear gaining weight?
- Maintain a weight lower than normal for your age, height, and genetic make up?
- Have irregular or no menstrual cycles (for women)?

If you answered "yes" to any of these questions, you may have an eating disorder. But, don't get alarmed. Continue reading as I describe in more detail the criteria for each eating disorder. If you see yourself in these descriptions, professional help will be appropriate. I will show you how to get such help later on.

**What is Anorexia Nervosa?**

Anorexia Nervosa, commonly referred to as "anorexia," is a medically recognized condition characterized by a person's refusal to maintain a normal weight, coupled with an intense fear of gaining weight and a distorted perception of one's body shape or size. What is so tragic about anorexia is that the people afflicted are deathly thin and yet they see themselves as overweight. Their refusal to eat makes treatment very difficult. For many, this refusal is not mere obstinacy. Rather it is a profound fear of eating that sets off biochemical reactions in their brain that ultimately prohibit eating. Eventually, their disease progresses so far that they cannot eat. It is no longer a matter of "will not." Treatment for anorexia very often requires hospitalization.

Here is a checklist of common signs and symptoms of Anorexia Nervosa:
- refusal to maintain weight at or above a minimally normal weight for height and age
- intense fear of gaining weight
- distorted body image
- loss of three consecutive menstrual cycles (females)
- dehydration
- constipation
- edema (water retention)
- abdominal bloating
- abdominal pain

## What is Bulimia Nervosa?

Bulimia Nervosa, also known as "bulimia," is quite different from anorexia. Bulimia is characterized by binge eating. Bulimic people experience a sense of lack of control when it comes to eating. They will binge eat and then they will engage in "compensatory behaviors", such as vomiting, using laxatives, fasting, or excessively exercising in an effort to avoid gaining weight. In other words, to "undo the binge". In addition, a bulimic's self-esteem is related to body shape and weight. She feels good about herself if she is thin (or at least the scale says so) and she feels self-loathing if she believes she is fat. A bulimic's world centers around food, dieting, bingeing, and weight.

Here is a checklist of some common signs and symptoms of Bulimia Nervosa:
- Repeated episodes of binge eating and purging
- Feeling out of control during a binge episode
- Purging, vomiting, using laxative, diet pills, diuretics, fasting or excessive exercise after a binge
- Frequent dieting
- Extreme concern about weight and body size

- Skin rash
- Pimples
- Swelling or tenderness in salivary glands
- Constipation
- Edema
- Bloating
- Frequent cavities
- Enamel erosion

## What is Binge Eating Disorder?

There is another eating disorder which is beginning to gain recognition. It is called Binge Eating Disorder (BED). It is not yet considered an officially diagnosed disorder. Further research is underway to see whether it warrants inclusion in the *Diagnostic and Statistical Manual of Mental Disorders* (the "DSM"), the "bible" of mental heath disorders. The DSM is the official reference for all diagnosable mental conditions.

BED is very much like bulimia except that the person suffering with this malady does not engage in compensatory behavior. BED is characterized by eating fast, feeling uncomfortably full, being out of touch with hunger, feeling depressed, guilty or ashamed.

Here is a checklist of some common signs and symptoms of Binge Eating Disorder:
- Frequent episodes of eating abnormally large amounts of food
- Frequent feelings of being unable to control one's eating
- Eating rapidly
- Eating large amounts of food when not hungry
- Eating alone because embarrassed
- Feelings of disgust, depression or guilt after overeating

### How Do You Know If You Have an Eating Disorder?

The above descriptions of anorexia, bulimia, and BED should give you a fair idea of whether or not you have an eating disorder. If you believe that you meet any of the criteria set forth above, I strongly urge you to seek professional help. In Part Three, I discuss in more detail how, when, and where to find help.

### Treating Eating Disorders

In general eating disorders can be effectively treated with psychotherapy. This can be done in a group setting or through individual sessions with a trained professional. In many cases, medication is also part of the treatment plan. A psychiatrist is the right person to talk to about medication. For others, the most effective treatment for an eating disorder is a combination of psychotherapy, medical attention and nutritional counseling. Psychotherapy will address both the symptoms and the underlying psychological issues. Nutritional counseling teaches healthy eating habits and food choices and is usually provided by a registered dietitian or nutritionist. The medical component includes physical examinations and medication evaluations. In general, treatment is usually out-patient and includes, individual, group and family therapy. Hospitalization maybe recommended for those who are suffering from a life threatening physical condition or when there is evidence of severe emotional disturbance. Part Three includes a partial list of treatment facilities that may be of use.

If you believe that you have an eating disorder, take this book with you when you go to your physician, psychiatrist or psychotherapist for an evaluation. Show them the descriptions above that describe you. In addition, I provided space for you to write down your reasons why you believe you may have an eating disorder. Use this space to organize your thoughts so you can present your concerns clearly to your medical or mental health provider. Then, allow them to make the necessary recommendations.

*Why I Believe I Have An Eating Disorder:*

_____

_____

_____

_____

_____

_____

_____

_____

If you need additional assistance, there is also help available through various associations and organizations. A list of such associations and organizations is offered in Part Three. Your physician and your local reference librarian can help with more.

## Why Do You Overeat?

"Doctor, why do I overeat?" is one of the most frequently asked questions in therapy. So often my patients feel like there is something wrong with them. They feel weak, evil, or bad. But, they are none of those things. Instead they are brave, strong, and troubled. All they do is overeat in response to stress, anxiety, and other uncomfortable feelings. What do you do? When things get overwhelming do you find yourself reaching for a candy bar, donut, or ice-cream, or whatever your "binge" food is? Why do you do this? The answer is simple—food works! It's fast. It's easy. It's available. It's legal. And for the moment, after you have eaten that candy bar, donut or ice-cream you feel better. You feel relief. That's why you do it. And that's why overeating is so hard to give up. Unfortunately, even though you momentarily feel better your problem is not solved and in the end you may feel worse because you berate yourself for having eaten on top of everything else.

To make matters even more difficult, you have to eat to stay alive. Unlike alcohol, cigarettes or recreational drugs which you can abstain from for the rest of your life and survive, you have to eat. At least three times a day, seven days a week, fifty two-weeks a year for as long as you are on this earth. If you abstain you die. For the troubled eater, each eating episode is a dilemma—*"what should I eat, how much, is what I am eating okay, will it make me fat, am I eating too much?"* and so on. It is a struggle every time.

Sound familiar? Feeling hopeless? I hope not! There is a way out. You will find out in Week 1 that the first step is to acknowledge that food is the way you cope with your emotions. No judgment. Just fact. This is what you do. Others smoke. Some drink. You eat. During Week 1 you will acknowledge this and make it "okay" and then find other ways to cope.

I would like you to meet Connie. Connie is an attractive professional woman in her early thirties. She has a successful career which carries a lot of responsibility. Connie is also sixty pounds overweight. When Connie describes her job she talks mostly about the pressure she feels and the demands on her time. She often complains about there not being enough hours in the day to get everything done that is expected of her. When Connie starts to feel overwhelmed she reaches for the candy jar which stands on her desk. There are days when that jar is empty before twelve o'clock. Connie is clearly overeating in response to the stress of her job. As Connie works her ways through this program she will learn about other ways to cope with her stress that don't involve reaching into that jar! The less she reaches for candy, the more weight she will lose. That's how this process works.

As a beginning, spend a few moments thinking about why you overeat. Use the space provided to write down your thoughts and insights. It will be interesting for you to come back to this section later and review what you have written so early in the process.

*Why I Overeat...*

_____

_____

_____

_____

_____

_____

_____

_____

## What Kind of Overeater Are You?

There are many types of overeaters. I will give a description of four types. See if you can find yourself in any of them. Knowing the kind of overeater you are will help enormously as you work your way into another way of eating.

### The Feeler

The first type of overeater we will look at is the Feeler. This is the person who eats in response to specific emotions or feelings. Since you have picked up this book, I expect you will find yourself in this description. The Feeler eats in response to emotions such as anxiety, boredom, conflict, depression, or insecurity. This eating is usually done in secret and feels rebellious. It's the "I'll show her. I'll eat this ice cream sandwich. That'll get her." By eating, the Feeler believes that she is managing her emotions and has a sense of relief afterwards.

### The Snacker

The second type of overeater is the Snacker. The Snacker is not physically hungry when she eats. Her eating is usually controlled and occurs in the late afternoon or evenings. It's not uncommon for the Snacker to eat in secret since she feels somewhat ashamed of eating again. Although unaware, the Snacker is eating emotionally if she is not genuinely hungry at the time she chooses to snack.

### The Grazer

The third type of overeater is the Grazer. A Grazer eats throughout day. There is no intense emotion as there is for the Feeler, rather just a vague sense of distress such as boredom. Grazers usually feel in control of their eating and don't usually eat very much food at any one time.

### The Binger

The fourth overeater is the Binger. The Binger eats large quantities of food in relatively short periods of time and generally feels a sense of being out of control. Feeling such as anger and frustration lead to binges more often than other emotions, such as depression.

Did you find yourself in any of these descriptions? Use the space below to records your impressions about the type of emotional overeater you are.

*I am a* _____ *Type Overeater Because…..*

_____

_____

_____

_____

_____

_____

_____

## How People Become Overeaters

How people become overeaters is an interesting question. Volumes of professional material are available to answer this provocative inquiry. For our purposes I will highlight four reasons for this behavior.

### Culture and Religion

For some, cultural traditions and religious practice contribute to the development of overeating as a behavior pattern. Food, its preparation as well as its consumption, plays an important role in the lives of many people. Think of our traditional Thanksgiving dinner. If you are like most people, your dinner table is filled with turkey, stuffing, cranberry sauces, breads, potatoes, pies, cakes, cookies, and so on. The list, like the meal, is endless. It is very common for Thanksgiving diners to overeat. Who can pass up all these delicacies?

Theresa is an excellent example of a person who learned to overeat because of cultural reasons. Theresa is an Italian-American. Her parents moved to the United States a few years before she was born. They brought with them Theresa's paternal grandmother. She lived with Theresa's family until her death at age 94. Theresa recalls fond memories of her home being filled with the smell of good old-fashioned Italian cooking. Every meal was a feast. Her grandmother took great delight in cooking and watching Theresa and her two siblings eat. Theresa was taught that food was love and so learned very early on to eat everything that was put in front of her. Theresa told me a story once about a time she tried to diet before her wedding. Her family, especially her grandmother, was so offended by her refusal to join them in hearty meals that she soon abandoned her weight loss efforts because of all the bad feelings she experienced.

Think back to your own cultural and religious upbringing. What role did food play? How important is food to your traditions and practices?

Do you have a habit of overeating during festive times? What about at times of sorrow? Is food part of your grief process? Use the space provided to reflect on your personal story.

### *My Traditions and Practices*

_____

_____

_____

_____

_____

_____

_____

_____

_____

_____

_____

### Childhood Issues

Another reason why people develop the habit of overeating can be traced to childhood issues. The issues that lead to this behavior vary from person to person but some of the more common ones are:

- **The Clean Your Plate Club.** You may remember this club. This was the club that did not allow you to have dessert, go out and play, watch television, or use the telephone until all the food on your plate is finished. Never mind that you were not hungry or that you did not like the food choices served. You had to finish everything, or else! By eating this way, you not only learned the habit of overeating but you also never learned to eat according to your own needs and preferences. Fortunately, this is a skill you will learn in the weeks to come.
- **There are Children Starving in Africa.** How many times did you hear this one? It might not have been Africa. It could have been

Europe or China or Southeast Asia. The feeling provoked by this statement was guilt. You were meant to feel guilty for not eating because others were not "as lucky as you" to have all this wonderful food. So what did you do? You ate it. Once again hunger and food preferences were not considered. And, once again the habit of overeating, the habit of eating outside of your hunger, was instilled.

- **Depression Era Babies.** Depression Era babies are people who were either born during the Great Depression or who were raised by people who experienced it. People who experienced the deprivation associated with that time in American history were taught to take food when it was served and to not waste any of it. Consequently, eating more when it was presented, even if not hungry, is a common behavior pattern that has led many to a weight problem.

Do you recognize any childhood issues that may have affected your relationship to food? Take a moment to look at the issue more closely before moving on.

*My Childhood Affected My Eating Habits in the Following Ways....*

_____

_____

_____

_____

_____

_____

_____

_____

_____

### Dieting or Restrictive Eating

Did you know that dieting actually makes you fat? It is true. The reason why diets make you fat is that a diet is usually followed by a period of overeating, sometimes even a full blown binge. The restriction and deprivation that diets cause set you up to rebound into food. What do I mean by this? I mean that when all you have eaten for a week is hard-boiled eggs, grapefruit and broiled fish, a pizza sure sounds good. So after a week or so of deprivation you treat yourself to some pizza. For most people, one slice does not cut it. Once they start on the pizza they keep going, either by eating more pizza or by eating more of other food. Either way, overeating occurs. In Week Four, we will explore the role diets have played in your weight struggle. For now, it is enough to consider the possibility that all your dieting and other forms of restrictive eating have actually caused you to overeat.

### Food Triggers

The final cause of overeating that we will look at is called Food Triggers. For some people certain foods trigger overeating. In some diet circles these foods are known as "red light" foods or "illegal" foods. Whatever their title, these foods cause people to eat more of them than they are hungry for. Some common trigger foods are: chocolate, potato chips (remember the old commercial "No one can eat just one!",) ice cream, French fries, and nuts. Do you have food triggers? Are there foods you feel you need to stay away from because you eat too much of them when they are present? Use the space below to list your trigger foods.

*My Food Triggers*

_____

_____

_____

_____

_____

_____

_____

_____

_____

_____

_____

Now that we have explored some of the more common causes of overeating, we can move onto another important topic that influences eating behavior.

### It is Also About Self-Esteem

This topic is one you may not have considered before. One you might not have included in your answer above. This one is a little bit more complicated than the others. This reason is about you—who you are, how you view yourself, how you feel about yourself. This reason is all about self-esteem.

What is self-esteem? Self-esteem is the level of regard we hold for ourselves. If we value ourselves highly, we take good care of ourselves in all circumstances of our lives. We have high self-esteem. On the other hand, if we hold ourselves in low regard we let external forces rule our lives. We have low self-esteem.

People who turn to food to cope generally have low self-esteem. By this I mean that the overeater does not value herself enough to want to take better care of herself. This is seen in many areas of her life—not just in her relationship to food. For example, she may not say no to someone who asks a favor of her when she is clearly unable to assist. Or, she may not go to her dentist or physician for an examination. Or, she may drink or smoke too much.

When you address self-esteem and start to value yourself more, you will start to take better care of yourself. As you take better care of yourself, you will find yourself choosing your foods more carefully. You will want to feel better and to feel better you will eat less and more healthfully. Over time, as your self-esteem goes up, your weight comes down.

Now for the tricky part. How do you build self-esteem? The answer is actually quite simple, although implementing it may not be so easy. The answer is "Do the tough stuff!" You know what I am talking about. It's the stuff you know you are "supposed" to do but you don't want to. For example, you just broke up with your boyfriend and you know you shouldn't call him but the urge is real strong. RESIST! Not calling him when that is the right thing for you to do builds self-esteem. It may not feel good in the moment, but the moment will pass and it will sure feel good later on when you're over him and you realize that you didn't make a fool of yourself calling him a hundred times a day! Here's another example. You have a report to write for work or school and you get invited to see a play. You know that you need to write the report and that going to the play will prevent you from finishing it. CHOOSING THE REPORT builds self-esteem. Again, it may not feel good in the moment, especially when you think of your friends enjoying the show, but it will feel great in the morning when you can hand in your report on time. That feeling of accomplishment builds self-esteem. Doing the tough stuff makes a difference.

Gerry, a 49 year old patient of mine, earned much of her self-esteem when she quit smoking. She said that quitting smoking was the hardest thing she ever did and now that it's done she can do anything! Now that's confidence. That's self-esteem!

You will see this in progress as you work on overcoming your emotional overeating. Each time you choose to do something other than eat, you build your self-esteem. Each small self-esteem success builds on the next. Over time, you will feel differently about yourself. You will care more about yourself and as a result you will take better care of yourself. This, my dear friend, is high self-esteem.

What is some of the "tough stuff" that you know you need to do and are not doing? Take a moment to think about this. Write down some of these things. Then, when you are ready, do them and see how much better you feel about yourself for having done them. Good luck!

*"Tough Stuff" I Know I Need To Do and Am Avoiding:*

_____

_____

_____

_____

_____

_____

_____

_____

_____

_____

## Eating and Weight are Just Symptoms

By now you may be thinking "when is she going to get to the part about losing weight? I bought this book to teach me how to stop overeating because I want to lose weight." Well, I have some bad news for you. This is not a diet book. Oh, you'll lose weight (if you truly have weight to lose) when you stop overeating, but not because of some scheme that you will find between these pages. The weight will come off when the underlying issues of why you overeat in the first place are resolved. You see eating and weight are just symptoms. They are not the problems. Just like you turn to food to relieve stress and anxiety because it works, you are overweight and/or focused on your weight because it works. It distracts you from the other things going on in your life that needs attention. For example, maybe you are in a bad marriage and it is too frightening to look at because then you might have to do something about it. Or, you are having trouble with a co-worker and are too afraid to confront him. Saying something such as "my husband is mean to me because I am fat. If I lose weight then he'll treat me better" puts all the focus on your weight and not where it belongs—on your husband's behavior. You know what to do if the problem is your weight—you go on another diet. But if the problem is your husband's behavior you don't know what to do (or you do and don't want to do it) so you avoid it.

Identifying these underlying issues will occur as you move through this program. We will discuss more about what are some of these underlying issues as we move along.

How are weight and eating issues just symptoms for you? Write your answer below.

*Weight and Eating are Just Symptoms for Me Because...*

_____

_____

_____

_____

_____

_____

### Why People Gain Weight

Let's take a moment to explore seven reasons, other than emotional overeating, for why people gain weight.

## Genetics.

The first reason is Genetics. You may not want to face this but weight is partially determined by heredity. There are about 200 different genes that play a role in weight issues. Take a look at your family tree. If you come from strong Germanic stock, you will never be a svelte ballerina. If you come from an Asian background, you will probably never be a football player. It is important to come to terms with what genes you have inherited and what body size is reasonable for you. This means getting real on what a healthy body for you will be. It does not mean giving up and giving in if you come from heavier genes. I have heard many people say "I'm big boned I'll never be skinny so why bother?" Sure you may never be skinny if you have large bones, but you can be healthy and lean for your frame.

## Age.

It is natural to gain weight as we get older. As we age our metabolic efficiency goes up. This means that it takes less energy to do things so we gain weight. In addition, our muscle mass decreases so we burn less calories moving around. Consequently, it is not reasonable to think you will weight the same at age 48 as you did at age 18. But you don't have to be overweight either!

## Culture, traditions and rituals.

This topic was explored earlier when we looked at some of the reasons how people become overeaters. If you haven't already done so, take a look at the rituals in your life and see if they are adding to your pounds. Remember to include the traditional coffee breaks so common in our offices today.

## Food Quantities.

Calories do count. If you eat more calories than your body needs to survive, you will gain weight. It's that simple. In the end, it makes little

difference if those excess calories come from protein or low-fat carbo-
hydrates, or even non-fat foods. If you eat more than your body needs,
you will gain weight.

### Food Choices.

Even if you feel that the quantities you are choosing are right, your
food choices may also be making you fat. Today's prepared food items
contain increased amounts of fat and sugar. These hidden ingredients
add considerable calories to your meal. So while you may not be eating
large quantities of food, your food choices maybe calorie dense in
which case you are taking in more calories than your body needs to
function and you gain weight. As an experiment, start reading the labels
of the food you choose. Notice the fat and calorie content. Become an
educated consumer. Know what you are eating so you can make wise
choices for yourself.

### Sedentary Lifestyle.

Did you know that today's technological advances lead to weight
gain? All the labor saving devices we enjoy such as power windows
and TV remote control cause us to gain weight. How you ask? It's
rather obvious if you think about it. All of our labor saving devices
have us moving less. If you are moving less you are using fewer calories. If you are using fewer calories but still consuming the same
amount as before your labor saving devices, you will gain weight.
Consider this. If you had to get up from your chair every time you
wanted to change television channels you would burn a few calories. A
pound of weight is equal to approximately 3,500 calories. So over time
those calories burned changing the channels would add up to lost
pounds. If you are just sitting there not moving, you are not using up
those 3,500 calories and your weight stay where it is or goes up
depending on how much you eat. How is our technology causing you
to gain weight? Are you gaining weight because you are less active?

Toby did. After Toby graduated college and started working as a computer programmer she started putting on weight. Active on her college track team, Toby stopped exercising when she started working. It wasn't long before the pounds crept up on her. The cause of Toby's weight gain is easy to spot. Is yours? Write your answers here.

*Sedentary Lifestyle and Technology are Making Me Fat by…*

_____

_____

_____

_____

_____

_____

_____

_____

**Lifestyle changes.**

Lifestyle changes such as getting married cause weight gain. A married person will gain an average of 42.5 pounds if unhappy and 18 pounds if happy! One reason experts suggest is that the decrease in intimacy in an unhappy marriage leads to an increase in food consumption. Another reason offered is that some spouses want their partners to be overweight so they present no threat to the marriage. Sharon gained weight after marrying Larry but not because she was unhappy. She gained weight because she stopped paying attention to her appearance. She figured that since she was married it didn't matter anymore. Does it matter to you? Does being in a relationship add weight to your body? Think about it.

Other lifestyle changes that contribute to weight gain include moving from a house with stairs to a ranch style house. Another is taking a sedentary job. Still another is carpooling to work instead of walking. Is your lifestyle contributing to a weight problem? If so what can you do to change it?

### My Lifestyle and My Weight

_____

_____

_____

_____

_____

_____

_____

_____

_____

_____

### Overeating is Learned Behavior

Another frequently asked question is "How did I get this way?" Or, in other words, "How did I start overeating in the first place?" My clinical experience and research has led me to the conclusion that overeating is a learned behavior. That somewhere in your history someone taught you to eat in response to situations that have nothing to do with hunger. You may not have to search far in your memory to see where this comes from. For example, how many times when you were a child did your parents offer you a lollipop to stop crying or an ice cream cone for a good report card? How many well-meaning mothers stick a bottle in their crying baby's mouth thinking their child is hungry when in fact she needs changing or holding? Are you starting to get the picture?

Now don't get me wrong. I am not here to blast mothers or fathers. Parents do the best they can given who they are and who their parents were. What I am saying is that when food is offered as a reward or pacifier, it sets up a lifetime pattern of turning to food for things other than hunger.

In addition, take a look at the eating habits of your parents, siblings, and friends. Do any of them eat in response to stress and anxiety? Do any of them reward themselves with a steak dinner after closing an important deal? How many of them are on diets? Take a moment to think about this. We are in many ways products of our environment. If your environment is filled with people who "abuse" food, chances are you will abuse it too. Again, this doesn't make you or them bad or evil. It's just what you and they do that is the problem.

The good news is that if overeating is learned behavior it can be unlearned. And, that is exactly what this journey is all about.

Where might you have learned this kind of behavior? Write your reflections in the space below.

### *I Learned To Overeat From:*

_____

_____

_____

_____

_____

_____

_____

_____

_____

_____

_____

### Overeating as Coping
Before we move on to how to stop overeating. Let's take another look at the idea that overeating is a coping mechanism.

What is coping? Coping is what you do when stuff happens. Good stuff. Not so good stuff. Down right awful stuff. It's accepting a compliment on a job well done. It's calling the plumber when the drain clogs. It's grieving when a relationship ends. It's responding appropriately to a situation when the situation arises.

Some of us don't cope so well. Some of us reject the compliment and believe that the person offering it is "just saying that to be nice", or, worse yet, "wants something." Some of us cry instead of using the phone when the drain clogs. Some of us sink into deep depressions that last for years when a relationship ends. Some of us eat to cope. Somehow eating that donut gives us the strength (or smarts) to do what we need to do or to avoid the things we need to do. Somehow eating a lot and often helps the pain of an ended relationship go away. Somehow food works, whether by distracting us from what's really going on, numbing us so we don't feel the pain, or fortifying us so we can do what we need to do. Food works. Fortunately, so do a lot of the things. Hang in there a bit longer with me and you'll see what "other things" I am talking about.

Diane shared with me a life changing insight about her relationship with food. It was during the Persian Gulf conflict and she was in her den watching the news. She could feel herself get more and more anxious as the reporters talked about the bombs that were dropped and the lives that were lost. As her anxiety started to get the best of her she got up and went into the kitchen. She toasted a bagel, spread butter on it, and brought it back to the den. She sat down and bit into the bagel. Instantly she felt better. She could feel the anxiety and fear leave her body. It was in that moment that Diane made her connection between food and feelings. Diane understood how she had been using food as a "tranquilizer" all her adult life. That moment was the catalyst for a lot of change and the beginning of the end of her using food to cope. Do you use food to cope? This a tough question. Think about it for a while. Use the space provided to start formulating your answer.

*How I Use Food To Cope:*

_____

_____

_____

_____

_____

_____

_____

Congratulations, you have just completed Part One of your journey to overcoming emotional overeating. If you have done the exercises along the way, you have learned a lot about yourself and your relationship to food. All that information will help you as you move through Part Two the actual 15 week program. Are you ready to start? Good for you! Let's go!

# PART TWO:

## 15-WEEKS TO OVERCOMING EMOTIONAL OVEREATING

Welcome! This is the Part you have been waiting for. If you jumped here with reading Part One, that's just fine. But, I strongly recommend that you do read it eventually. It lays the foundation for the techniques offered later. But for now, since you are here, let's get going!

To get you started, I want to outline my suggestions of how best to approach this material. As you know the program is divided into 15 week segments. I recommend that you spend a full week on each segment. Begin by reading the week's material. Then go back and over the course of the week do the exercises, quizzes, and assignments as they present themselves. At the end of the week, if you feel that you have a good grasp of the ideas and insights presented, move forward to the next week. If you feel stuck or unsure, do the week again and move on when you feel ready. This is not a race. You are making changes in your relationship with food that will last a lifetime, so take your time to really understand the material. It will certainly be worth your while. You may want to keep a journal during this time. You can use the journal to record your thoughts, feelings, and insights as you move along. In the Workbook in Part Four is a journal. You can use that one or start one of your own. That having been said, it's time to begin. You are now ready to start Week One. Good luck and have fun!

# WEEK ONE:

## Acknowledging That You Are An Emotional Eater

Week One: Acknowledging That You Are an Emotional Eater

This week is about acknowledging that you are an emotional eater and noticing how that affects your life. It is important when you start a journey such as this one to know not only where you are going but also where are right now. To get you off to a good beginning, I included a quiz to help you understand the extent to which you eat in response to emotions. For each emotion listed, indicate how strong your need to eat in response is.

## Emotions Quiz Number One

| | None | Some | Moderate | Strong | Extreme |
|---|---|---|---|---|---|
| Anger | | | | | |
| Blue | | | | | |
| Bored | | | | | |
| Confused | | | | | |
| Discouraged | | | | | |
| Edgy | | | | | |
| Excited | | | | | |
| Frustrated | | | | | |
| Furious | | | | | |
| Happy | | | | | |
| Guilty | | | | | |
| Helpless | | | | | |
| Inadequate | | | | | |
| Irritated | | | | | |
| Jealous | | | | | |
| Jittery | | | | | |
| Lonely | | | | | |
| Loved | | | | | |
| Nervous | | | | | |
| Resentful | | | | | |
| Sad | | | | | |
| Scared | | | | | |
| Successful | | | | | |
| Tired | | | | | |
| Uneasy | | | | | |

## Scoring the Quiz

To score the quiz, give yourself the points indicated for each column. Column 1: 0 points; Column 2: 1 points; Column 3: 2 points; Column 4: 3 points; Column 5: 4 points. Now add up your scores. A score of 0-25 means you are a mild emotional eater. A score of 25-50 means you do considerable emotional eating. A score of 50-100 means you may have a serious emotional eating problem. What score did you get? Put your score here _____. As you move through the upcoming weeks, it might be interesting for you to come back to this quiz and take it again. I have a feeling that over time your scores will go down.

### What Being an Emotional Eater Really Means

If you are an emotional eater, it means that you have chosen to use food to nurture yourself. You have chosen to use food to make yourself feel better. In the weeks to come you will learn how to self- nurture without using food. To begin this part of your journey we will take a look at your self-nurturing attitudes and behaviors. An attitude is a perspective you have on something. For our purposes we will be focusing on your attitudes towards yourself and food. Specifically, learning to like yourself and to break destructive thinking habits. A behavior is an action you take in a particular circumstance. Some of the behaviors we will be looking at include taking your life off hold and finding substitutes for misusing food. To get the ball rolling, answer the following questions. Be as honest with yourself as you can. You owe it to yourself.

### My Attitudes and Behaviors

- My attitude towards myself can best as described as:

_____

_____

_____

_____

_____

- My attitude towards food can best be described as:

_____

_____

_____

_____

- If I liked myself I would:

  _____
  _____
  _____
  _____
  _____

- If I had a healthy relationship with food I would:

  _____
  _____
  _____
  _____
  _____

- The following thoughts about myself run through my head:

  _____
  _____
  _____
  _____
  _____

- The following thoughts about food run through my head:

  _____
  _____
  _____
  _____
  _____

- I am a positive thinker. True or False? _____

- I am optimistic. True or False? _____

• I am keeping my life on hold by:

_____

_____

_____

_____

_____

• Instead of eating when I am upset, I could do the following:

_____

_____

_____

_____

_____

When Laura did this exercise she realized that she has a "love/hate" relationship with food. She loves how food tastes but hates how overeating makes her feel about herself. She tends to beat herself up emotionally after eating too much and that lowers her self-esteem. Laura has come to understand that by dealing directly with her feelings she actually builds up her self-esteem and consequently is practicing doing so everyday.

So, you have come to end of Week One. How do you feel? What did you learn about yourself? Put your thoughts and reflections below.

**My First Week**

_____

_____

_____

_____

_____

_____

# Week Two:

## Assessing Your Readiness To Change The Way You Live Your Life

Week Two: Assessing Your Readiness to Change The Way You Live Your Life

Congratulations! You completed Week One and are now ready to move on. Or are you? Week Two is about deciding whether or not you are actually ready to do the things you need to do to overcome emotional overeating. Remember this is a lifestyle change. Up until now you have chosen to use food to cope. If you are going to conquer this problem once and for all this behavior will have to stop. You will no longer exercise the option of using food to cope. You will chose to live your life differently so that you have other skills at your disposal to cope with life.

To assess your readiness to change the way you live your life, answer True or False to the following 5 questions. Circle your response.

Question 1. I am willing to control my emotional eating tendencies. True/False.

Question 2. My reasons for wanting to lose weight are realistic, permanent, and based on what I want for myself not others. True/False.

Question 3. Currently there are no major upheavals in my life that could prevent me from devoting time and energy to this process. True/False.

Question 4. The goals I set for myself are realistic given who I am and what I am capable of.
True/False.

Question 5. I am ready to make a commitment to change how I live my life.
True/False.

If you answered true to these questions, you are ready to move on. If you did not, you may want to wait until the answers are all true. Let's take a look at each question, to see what it was really getting at.

**Question 1: "I am willing to control my emotional eating tendencies."**
This question is aimed at assessing your willingness to change. To change you must be willing. If you resist this process nothing will be different and you are just wasting your time trying. So really take a good look at yourself. Assess your willingness honestly. If you find that you are not willing, that's okay. Put this book down for a while. Pick it up again later when your willingness is more apparent. Take a moment to reflect on your current state of willingness. You can use the space provided to write your thoughts.

### My Willingness

_____

_____

_____

_____

_____

_____

**Question 2:** "My reasons for wanting to lose weight are realistic, permanent, and based on what I want for myself not others."

Most of you came to this program because you want to lose weight. You are carrying extra weight because you eat too much. You eat too much because you eat in response to emotions. If you are like most of my patients, you are hoping that once you conquer your emotional overeating problem, you will lose weight. If you are carrying extra weight because of the extra food you are eating in response to your emotions, you will lose weight once you stop that behavior. Wanting to lose weight can be a good goal for yourself if your reasons for doing so are the "right" ones. The "right" reasons include health, a desire for an improved lifestyle and increased self-esteem. Some "wrong" reasons are because your husband thinks you are fat or because your 20th high school reunion is next month or because you think losing weight will solve your other problems. What are your reasons for losing weight? Are they realistic? Aimed at long-lasting results and permanent change? Are they for you or for someone else? Use the space provided to sort through your reasons.

**My Reasons For Losing Weight Include:**

_____
_____
_____
_____
_____
_____
_____

What did you discover? Can you answer true to Question 2?

**Question 3:** "Currently, there are no major upheavals in my life that could prevent me from devoting time and energy to this process."

To be successful at this program, you will have to be available to do the work. You will need time, energy, and dedication. If you are currently involved in other ventures that will distract you from this process, this may not be the best time for you to tackle this problem. This is nothing wrong with postponing this program until a time when you are more available. So, if you are in the process of moving or starting a new job or getting divorced, you may want to wait. But, I caution you there will never be a perfect time to do this program. Life happens. In fact this book and this program is about life. It's about coping with life in a constructive manner. Nancy made the choice to wait a few months before beginning this program. When Nancy was first introduced to this program she was studying for the bar exam. Studying for that exam is tough and required her undivided attention. Together we decided that she would be better off waiting until the exam was finished before starting Week One. Making that decision postponed her start by six weeks. But it was well worth the wait because once she got started, Nancy worked hard to make significant changes in her relationship with food. And she passed her exam to boot!

Take a look at your life right now. Are thing pretty steady for you right now? Or are things chaotic? Is this a good time for you to devote yourself to your healing or would waiting be better? Decide below.

**Now or Later?**

_____

_____

_____

_____

_____

_____

Question 4: " The goals I set for myself are realistic given who I am and what I am capable of."

This question is related to Question 2 which explored your reasons for wanting to lose weight. This question's focus is a bit more general and wonders whether you are able to set realistic goals for yourself. Think about some of the goals you have set for yourself in your life, were they realistic? Did you succeed? You will be setting goals for yourself during this program. The most obvious goal will be doing each week's material. Are you ready? Are you willing? Are you able? Think about it.

### My Goal Setting History

_____

_____

_____

_____

_____

_____

_____

_____

_____

_____

_____

Question 5: "I am ready to make a commitment to change how I live my life."

Finally we come to the last question. As I mentioned above, this process will take time, energy, and dedication. Believe me this process is worth it. Once you get the hang of living your life differently, you will never want to go back to your old ways. Your life will run more smoothly and will bring you more joy. Sound good? I hope so. With these thoughts in mind, assess your level of commitment. What do you think?

### I am Committed to:

_____

_____

_____

_____

_____

_____

_____

_____

_____

_____

_____

Now that we have explored each question in depth, have your answers changed? Are you more or less ready to begin? Reflect on what you have learned here.

### My Reflections on My Readiness

_____

_____

_____

_____

# WEEK THREE:

## Your Diet And Weight History

Week Three: Your Diet and Weight History

Remember in Week One we discussed the importance of knowing where you are starting from to know where you are going? Well, we are going to apply that same principle this week when we take a long hard look at your diet and weight history. It is important to take the time to do this review because your diet and weight history will offer a lot of information about what your body (and you!) have been through, what a healthy weight for you could be, and how you and your body respond to diets and weight loss regimes.

To begin, look at your dieting history. Make a list of all the diets you were ever on, when you were on them, how much weight you lost, how long you kept the weight off, how much you regained, and when you regained it. We will be referring back to your list in a week to come. Take your time doing this. Be as thorough as possible. If you start to feel discouraged because of all your previous attempts, try to think about your diet experience in another way. Try to look at your experience as evidence of your commitment to be healthy and your personal qualities of persistence and tenacity. They will come in handy as you work to change your life through this 15-week program.

## *My Dieting History*

_____

_____

_____

_____

_____

_____

_____

_____

Next look at your weight history. Using the chronology set forth below, fill in your weights to the best of your recollection. Some of my patients find that looking at old photographs helps them approximate their weight at various times in their life.

## *My Weight Chronology*

Birth:

Age 5:

Age 13:

High School Graduation:

Age 20:

Wedding Day:

Age 30:

Age 35:

Age 40:

Age 50:

Today:

If you are like most of my patients, you have dieted yourself down to some pretty low weights. And if you are like them, you didn't stay there very long. I call those low weights "artificial" weights. You were artificially thin at those moments of your life. Not naturally slim. Natural slimness, the weight that suits your body best, is the weight we are after. Consider your weight history. Of all the weights you have been, what was your "best" weight? I define "best" weight as the weight that you maintained for a significant amount of time, that you felt good at, and that was relatively easy to achieve. This weight will most likely be your natural weight and the weight you achieve when you have healed your emotional eating behavior. What is your "best" weight? Write it down here _____.

Tiffany, age 28, and about 5 foot 6 inches, finally let go of her fantasy size "0" when she acknowledged that the only way she could maintain a size "0" was to eat no fat in her diet and to run at least 6 miles a day. She started by adding some fat back into her diet. She allowed herself some mayonnaise on her sandwiches and dressing on her salads. She noticed that adding that extra fat back made her feel physically better. She was less edgy, more energized and slept better. After a few weeks she cut down on her running. Running every other day for 2 to 3 miles. She is now a healthy and happy size 6 and looks and feels better than ever!

Are you ready to give up fantasy dieting? Are you ready to give up fantasy weights? Fantasy sizes? Are you willing to get real? For some of you these may be challenging questions. If you always dreamed of being a "perfect size 10", but you were only a size 10 once in your life and that was when you were a freshman in college it may be time to give up that fantasy size and get real. Reflect for a while on these questions, and write your (honest!) answers below.

*Getting Real*

_____

_____

_____

# WEEK FOUR:

## Admitting That Diets Don't Work

Week Four: Admitting that Diets Don't Work

I am about to tell you something you probably don't want to hear but that you already know in your heart to be true…. DIETS DON'T WORK! Realize that this is actually good news. Never again will you have to:

- Get weighed in anywhere
- Pay money to a weight loss program by the pound, the day, the week, the whatever
- Weigh your food
- Count calories
- Calculate fat grams
- Calculate carbohydrate grams
- Check off little boxes on a food chart
- Check off big boxes on a food chart
- Eat pre-packaged foods
- Eat foods that you hate but that are "good" for you
- Watch others enjoy a delicious meal while you munch on carrots
- Drink another liquid potion
- Pretend you are not hungry when you are
- Feel "bad" when you have eaten something gooey, sweet, fried, or whatever your "vice" may have been
- Feel deprived of the good things in life

## Why Diets Don't Work in The Long Run

For you those days are now over. I say good-bye and good ridden to them! Who needs them? Who needs all that deprivation? No one, including you. If you would prefer to enjoy life, to eat what you want when you want it, to truly taste food rather than gobble it down guilt fully over the kitchen sink, then give up diets once and for all! You see diets cause us all to do those things. Diets teach us that we are bad; that we do not know how to feed ourselves; and, that we do not know how to take care of ourselves. They set us up for failure and failure leads to bad feelings and bad feelings lead to overeating. So the cycle continues.

If diets worked you'd be thin now and you wouldn't have picked up this book. Sure, for the moment you are on a diet it works. You do lose weight. But, and this is a big but, you don't keep the weight off. Statistics tell us that only 5 to 10% of the people who lose weight on a diet keep it off. The rest regain their lost weight and then some. That's what makes the diet business a multi-billion dollar business. We keep going on diet after diet after diet.

Some people, maybe you, have abandoned diets. They have joined the "diets don't work" bandwagon, but they have not abandoned the diet mentality. Instead of counting calories, they are counting fat grams. Instead of keeping a food diary they are keeping exercise logs. Instead of restricting high-fat foods, they are gorging themselves on fat-free foods and artificially sweetened foods. Interestingly, we as a population are fatter now than before the advent of fat-free and the consumption of sugar has increased since the little pink packages first garnished our tables. Why, you may ask? The answer is quite simple. Fat-free foods are not calorie free foods. People erroneously believe that they can eat as much fat-free food as they want since it's fat free. Wrong! Wrong! Wrong! Next time you are in the supermarket, check the labels. You will see that many, if not most, of the fat-free products are higher in sugar and calories than their fat-free counterparts. Furthermore, artificial sweeteners actually make us crave sugar more than sugar does. Because artificial sweeteners are just that -artificial- they do not meet our natural cravings for sweets. They may fool us but they do not fool our brains. As we deny ourselves sugar, our brain hungers for more of it. Drinking lots of diet soft drinks can actually lead to a sugar binge. It is better to eat (and enjoy!) a piece of real, creamy, milk chocolate than to try to kid yourself with a make-believe candy bar. You'll be satisfied with less of the real thing and won't go grazing for more food later.

Another little known fact. Did you know that the best way to gain weight is to go on a diet? It's true. Over time diets cause our metabolisms to slow down. Thus it takes less and less food to meet our bodies' needs. Consequently, if you eat "like a normal person" you will in fact be eating too much for your metabolism and you will gain weight. That's why you are probably fatter today than you were when you went on your first diet. Sarah sure is. Sarah went on her first diet at age 15. At that time she was in junior high school and was about ten pounds overweight. The diet was successful and Sarah lost the ten pounds. In her senior year of high school she had put on some weight and wanted to diet it off before her prom. This time she had 18 pounds to lose. The 10 she lost a few years prior and 8 more. She went on the same diet but this time only lost 6 pounds. For the next 22 years, Sarah went on and off diets until her weight climbed to over 200 pounds. Sadly, she admitted to herself that if she never dieted in the first place and lived a lifestyle filled with exercise and other good habits she would be thinner and healthier today. Fortunately for Sarah, she found this program and is learning that very lifestyle today.

Using your dieting history exercise from Week Three, answer the following questions:

Question 1: Did dieting help you successfully lose weight and keep it off? Why or why not?

_____

_____

_____

_____

_____

Question 2: Were each of your dieting episodes followed by weight gain? If so, how much?

_____

_____

_____

_____

_____

Question 3: Were you hungry on your diets? And if so, did your hunger cause you to overeat?

_____

_____

_____

_____

_____

Question 4: Did you "cheat" when you were dieting? If so, what did you cheat on and how did your cheating affect your dieting?

_____

_____

_____

_____

_____

Question 5: What have you learned about dieting and weight loss by doing these exercises and answering these questions?

_____

_____

_____

_____

_____

## What Works

I hope that I have convinced you never to diet again. I know that for many of my patients the idea of never dieting again is frightening. Up until now, it has been their only hope to happiness and here I am saying to give it up! It's a frightening proposition. I know that. I understand. So go slowly. Remember nothing I write is intended to push you or to scare you. Go at your own rate. Incorporate my thoughts, ideas and suggestions into your life at a rate that feels comfortable to you. Remember there is no such thing as failure. This is a process. I am more concerned with the general directions you are going in, rather than how fast you get there.

So, if diets don't work. What does? Listening to your body and meeting its needs accordingly works. I hear those gasps again! I also hear comments such as "How can I trust my body, just look at it!" "If I trust my body I'll get even fatter." "If I trust my body, I'll never be thin." My question to you is " How can you not trust your body?" Take a minute and think about your body. Think about what it does in an ordinary day. Think about how it keep your lungs breathing and your heart pumping. Think about how it moves you in the world. How it solves problems for you. Think about the millions of cells that fight off disease. How can a body so intricate, so ingenuous, so powerful not be trustworthy? And more important how can a body not know what it needs? The problem is that we have became so used to listen outside ourselves for messages on what to eat, when to eat and how much to eat that we have lost track of our own body's messages. Listen closely and you will hear them. Look at a toddler. If left on her own over a period of a few days or a week, the toddler will naturally choose food that meets her physiological needs. But unfortunately well meaning parents or grandparents panic when all they see their beloved child eat is potato chips or cookies that they start to "force feed" strained peas and carrots or cereal. Yuck! We, as children, learn very early not to listen to our internal messages.

Society also gives us these messages. It seems as if everyday there is another report telling us what to eat and what not to eat. First eggs are bad. Now they are not so bad. Eat shrimp, don't eat shrimp. Milk is good, milk is bad. And so on. Magazines offer a new diet each month. You cannot escape the headlines while standing at the checkout counter: "Ten Days to a Perfect Body" or "Junk Food Forever Diet" or "Eat only Chocolate and Lose Weight". You have seen them. You know. Take a trip to your local bookstore and peruse the health section, the diet section and the magazines section and you will see what I mean. It can be confusing and overwhelming. It makes some people give up. Please don't give up! Give your weight loss efforts one more chance by trying the method I am offering.

Some of what I will share with you may run contrary to what you have heard about getting thin and staying thin. If you hang in there you will see that these ideas work.

To get a better understanding of the confusing information you received over the years about dieting and weight loss, think of the contrary messages you received about nutrition, diet and weight loss. What were you told? From whom did you receive these messages? Jot some of them down in the space below.

*Conflicting Messages I Received About Nutrition, Diet and Weight Loss*

_____

_____

_____

_____

_____

_____

_____

_____

_____

So, are you ready to give up dieting forever? Are you ready to accept that permanent weight loss comes only from changing your lifestyle and not from some diet found in the pages of a magazine? I hope so. Record your thoughts here and then you will be ready to move on to Week Five.

*My Final Thoughts on Dieting and Weight Loss*

_____

_____

_____

_____

_____

_____

_____

_____

_____

# Week Five:

## Accepting Your Body And Your Weight For Now

Week Five: Accepting Your Body and Your Weight For Now

Welcome to Week Five. This week we will address a very important issue that maybe difficult for you to do. The task for this week is accepting your body and weight now—whatever it is. I understand that you may hate the way you look now. You do not want to accept your current weight because you are afraid that if you accept your current weight it will never change. Fortunately nothing could be further from the truth. You need to accept who you are now before you can become the person you want to be. Before you can make the changes you want to make you need to know that you are okay just the way you are. Otherwise you are at war with yourself. As we know from real war, no one ever truly wins. Accepting your weight now does not mean you have to like it. Nor does it mean that you have to stay at this weight. It does mean that you won't fight yourself anymore about it. Once you do that you will feel a sense of inner calmness, some call it relief, and then you can begin the process of change.

What are your thoughts and feelings about the idea of accepting your weight right now. Write them down here:

*How I Feel About Accepting My Body and Weight Now:*

_____

_____

_____

_____

_____

_____

Here's some help in accepting your weight right now. I call this exercise the *Magic Gas Exercise*. Imagine for a moment that the atmosphere is suddenly filled with a gas that makes it impossible for you to ever gain or lose an ounce of weight. It does not matter if you eat a pound of chocolate or celery everyday your weight will not budge. It also wouldn't matter whether you sat on the couch all day watching soap operas or play in a tennis tournament. Your weight would never change. How do you feel about this? Are you excited or frightened? Are you saying "Let me lose twenty pounds and then fill the atmosphere with this magic gas?" Take some time to think about this. What would you do with yourself if food, weight, diet and exercise were no longer an issue? Would you still go to the gym? Would you still count fat grams? How would your life change? Or would it even change? Record your thoughts here.

*Magic Gas Exercise*

_____

_____

_____

_____

_____

_____

_____

_____

Did this exercise initially fill you with horror? Relief? Peace? What would you do with your time if diet and weight issues were forever removed from you life? Would you take up skiing? Painting? Go back to school? Watch old movies all day? Put your ideas here.

*What I Would Do If Food and Weight Were Not an Issue:*

_____

_____

_____

_____

_____

_____

_____

Now I want to pose another question to you—Why aren't you doing those things now? Is your immediate response that you are too fat? If you are willing to be truthful with yourself, that is not the real answer. The real answer lies somewhere else. It lies in fears, insecurities, and anxieties. It is only when you conquer those fears, insecurities and anxieties that the weight comes off. Live your life as if you were thin and you will become thin. Wait to live your life until you are thin and you'll stay fat. That is how it really works. Bonnie is a terrific example of someone who stopped using fat as an excuse and started living. Bonnie always wanted to be a school teacher but felt that because of her size the students wouldn't take her seriously. Bonnie was using being fat as a reason not to get her teaching credential. I told Bonnie that if she wanted her students to take her seriously, she needed to take herself seriously. So, Bonnie and I did some work in therapy around this issue. After a while, Bonnie developed the self-confidence to apply for her teaching certificate. She got it and today is living her life's dream as a fourth grade teacher.

What are some of the things you would do if weight were no longer an issue? Make your (very long) list below.

*What I Would Do If Weight Were No Longer An Issue*

_____

_____

_____

_____

_____

_____

_____

_____

_____

Now do one of them!

# WEEK SIX:

## Getting Rid Of The Scale

Week Six: Getting Rid of the Scale

The next step is to stop weighing yourself. Throw away your scale (or if you can't do that yet, put it away and throw it out later when you feel more confident.)

Throwing out your scale is not easy. What I am suggesting you do is to remove your most invested possession. What do I mean by "invested?" Well, think about it. You have a lot of your emotional well-being wrapped up in the scale. If you get on it in the morning and it says something you like, you smile and go about your day feeling happy, confident and in charge! But, if the scale says something you don't like that same day is spent in misery, self-hatred and anger. And chances are you will eat and eat and eat because "what you are doing doesn't work anyway" or "why bother" or "I'll start tomorrow" or "I am angry and when I am angry I eat" or…you can fill in the rest for yourself.

When I counsel patients who struggle with the scale issue, I help them to see the uselessness of stepping on the scale. I ask them to imagine themselves getting on the scale and seeing their ideal weight. They feel great. Then I ask them to imagine the scale is broken or their spouse kicked it off balance or their cat played with that little wheel that adjusts the zero or another contrived situation whereby the scale will be off and not register the correct weight. Now I have them imagine that they got back on the scale and now it says a number they don't like. Now they are miserable and all that happened is the scale got out of whack. Nothing else changed and yet their day is ruined.

So, I suggest you toss it. If you cannot bear to toss it, then hide it. Don't want to do that then paste your ideal weight over the numbers on the scale so that each time you step in it you see what you want to see! That's what Brenda did. Brenda's healthy ideal weight is 144 so she wrote that number on an index card and taped it to her scale. Seeing that number inspired her to work diligently on her week's assignments and made significant progress on her emotional eating problem.

Now I realize that for some of you the notion of removing your scale is terrorizing. You feel that if you don't have a scale to monitor yourself you will just keep getting fatter and fatter and fatter. Actually, the contrary is more likely occur. You will find as you apply the ideas in this program (including getting rid of the scale) you will lose weight. Use your clothes and your mirror to tell you how you are doing instead of the scale. And here's an additional note, don't pay attention to dress size either. One manufacturer's fourteen is another's ten. Just focus on what feels comfortable and makes you feel great about yourself.

I am going to give you two exercises to complete this week. The first has to do with getting rid of your scale and the second is about learning to assess your progress without it. Let's begin with the first exercise.

### Getting Rid of the Scale
**Part One: How Do You Feel About Your Scale**
In the space provided describe your feelings about your scale. Do you have a love/hate relationship with it such that you love it when it shows a low weight and hate it when it shows a high weight? Or, are you indifferent and

it's just another piece of furniture? Or, maybe you are one of the lucky ones who doesn't own a scale!

_____

_____

_____

_____

_____

_____

_____

How often do you weigh yourself? Does that work for you? If so, how?

_____

_____

_____

_____

_____

_____

_____

What about the scale at the doctor's office? Did you ever ask not to be weighed? Or turn your back to the scale if she insists?

_____

_____

_____

_____

_____

_____

_____

_____

**Part Two: How Do You Feel About Getting Rid of the Scale?**
Now describe how you feel about the prospect of getting rid of the scale. Do you feel anxious? Afraid that if you don't weigh yourself you will gain a lot of weight? Relieved?

_____

_____

_____

_____

_____

_____

_____

_____

_____

**Part Three: Getting Rid of the Scale**
Now comes your moment of truth. It's time to get rid of the scale. What are you going to do with it? Throw it out? Donate it to Goodwill? Hide it? Paste your "best" weight over the numbers?

_____

_____

_____

_____

_____

_____

_____

_____

_____

Well done! You did it! How do you feel? You are really making progress. I hope you can congratulate yourself for all your hard work so far. Okay, so now you are ready for the second exercise of the week, "New Measurements of Success."

## New Measurements of Success

Since you have gotten rid of your scale, it's time to figure out other ways to measure your health and your weight. Here are some of the ways my patients have come up with. You can use their ideas or come up with something on your own.

*New Measurements of Success*
- How clothing fits
- Using a favorite belt
- Better sleep
- Clearer skin
- Healthier nails
- Shinier hair
- How rings and other jewelry fit
- More energy
- Happier attitude
- More positive outlook

What will your new measurements of success be? Write them down here.

Before you get ready to move on to Week Seven, I want to address in general how a person can learn to stop overeating. Remember overeating is a learned response so that means it can be unlearned.

## How to Stop Overeating

So, just how do you stop overeating? The answer lies with understanding why you overeat and learning to get in touch with yourself and your true hunger. Let me explain.

There are two types of hunger: physical hunger and psychological hunger (also known as emotional hunger.) Physical hunger is what alerts you to your body's needs. It is the signal that tells you when to eat, what to eat and how much to eat. It is stomach grumbles, lightheadedness, irritability or headaches. Its signal is different for each person. If you listen it will guide you to your natural, healthy weight.

Psychological or emotional hunger is everything else! It is all the other times you eat that have nothing to do with physical hunger. For example, you come home from work at four o'clock in the afternoon and head straight for the refrigerator (even though you ate a full lunch at two o'clock and are not the least bit physically hungry). Or it is eight o'clock and you are watching television and you are mindlessly munching on chips. Or, it is midnight and you are at your computer and you need a break so you get some ice cream. It is also when you continue eating at a meal even though you are physically full. In each of these occasions, something else is operating other than true physical hunger. Finding out what that something else is part of the strategy for overcoming overeating. In the weeks ahead you will become an expert at this new skill.

We are now ready to continue to Week Seven. If you feel confident that you succeeded with the material and exercises in Week Six, keep going. If not, do some more work here and continue when you are ready.

# WEEK SEVEN:

## Making Food Conscious ~ Using Your Food Awareness Inventory

Week Seven: Making Food Conscious ~ Using Your Food Awareness Inventory

You are just about at the half way mark of your recovery program. So far you have uncovered a lot of valuable information about yourself, your dieting history, and your relationship with food. This week marks the beginning of further investigation of your relationship with food and the beginning of the changes in your lifestyle.

For this week, you will be keeping an eating record. I call this record your Food Awareness Inventory. The purpose of keeping the inventory is to gather information about your food patterns so that you can make more deliberate decisions regarding your eating.

Part Four, *The Do You Use Food To Cope Workbook*, contains your Food Awareness Inventory. It is set up for seven days. Feel free to complete the inventory directly in the Workbook or make copies of it for you to carry with you throughout the week.

When you turn to the Inventory you will notice that it contains space for you to make notations about the day of the week, the time you eat, the food or beverage you consume, the location you are at when you eat or drink and any other activities you may be engaged in at the same time. Complete the Inventory as best you can. At the end of the Inventory is some additional space for you to analyze what you observed about your eating habits over the course of the week. When you have completed the Inventory and Analysis return to this section to continue.

Now we are going to get a bit more specific about assessing your habits. Complete the chart below to get a better idea of your eating habits.

### *Assess The Number of Times You Ate:*

Before noon: _____

Between noon and 6pm: _____

Between 6pm and Midnight: _____

After midnight: _____

Other times: _____

At a Table:_____

In a Restaurant: _____

In the kitchen: _____

At your desk: _____

In your car: _____

Standing up over the sink: _____

Lying on sofa: _____

Lying in Bed: _____

Other places: _____

Sweets: _____

Meat: _____

Poultry: _____

Fish or Seafood: _____

Dairy Products: _____

Salty Foods: _____

Fruits: _____

Vegetables: _____
Other foods: _____

So, what have you learned? Barbara was surprised to see how many times she ate at her desk. She always considered it a "food-free" zone because she ate her meals in the office cafeteria. Keeping her Food Awareness Inventory showed her how much food she was actually eating while working. When Barbara made a conscious effort to eat less often at her desk she started losing weight. What have you noticed about your habits? What needs to be changed? Use the space provided to answer these questions.

### *My Eating Habits*

_____

_____

_____

_____

_____

_____

_____

_____

_____

Your assessment will be used later on as you move through the program.

If you feel satisfied that you understand your eating habits better and feel aware of the choices you are making, proceed to Week Eight where we will add an additional component to your Food Awareness Inventory.

# WEEK EIGHT:

## Relating To Your Emotions ~ Using Your Emotion Awareness Inventory

Week Eight: Relating to Your Emotions ~ Using Your Emotion Awareness Inventory

Remember the quiz you took in Week One? Now is the time to review your answers because this week we will be focusing on getting a better understanding of exactly how you respond to your emotions with food. To facilitate your understanding you will be completing another Inventory. This one is called Your Emotion Awareness Inventory. You will find it in the Workbook in Part Four, too. When completing this Inventory you will be recording the day of the week, the time you eat, the food and beverage you consume and the feeling or mood you are in when you were eating. As with the Food Awareness Inventory, there is space provided for you to do an initial analysis of your observations. When you have finished the inventory and the analysis, return to this section for further assessment.

It's time to take another quiz. This one is similar to the quiz in Week One, except this time you will be focused on the actual number of times you ate in response to a particular feeling or mood.

## *Emotions Quiz Number 2*

For each emotion, feeling, or mood listed below, write down the number of times over the course of this week that you ate when you felt it.

Anger: _____

Blue: _____

Bored: _____

Confused: _____

Discouraged: _____

Edgy: _____

Excited: _____

Frustrated: _____

Furious: _____

Happy: _____

Guilty: _____

Helpless: _____

Irritated: _____

Jealous: _____

Jittery: _____

Lonely: _____

Loved: _____

Nervous: _____

Resentful: _____

Sad: _____

Scared: _____

Successful: _____

Tired: _____

Uneasy: _____

Other: _____

Which emotion had the highest number? Are you noticing a pattern? Do negative emotions trigger you? Positive ones? Do you eat when you are tired? Bored? Angry? Put your insights here.

### *My Emotional Eating Patterns*

_____

_____

_____

_____

_____

_____

_____

_____

Now that you are becoming aware of your emotional eating patterns you are starting to create a choice for yourself. From now on, each time you feel an emotion that in the past led you to food, you have a choice. You can eat if you want to or not. Each time you choose not to eat in response to an emotion you move yourself closer to healing this problem once and for all.

Your thinking plays a major role in how your feel. What you tell yourself about a particular event, person, or circumstance can make the difference between feeling good and feeling bad. In clinical circles we refer to this process as the "antecedent, thought, emotion" cycle. For example, let's say you are preparing for a flight on an airplane. That's the antecedent. Then you think "the plane might crash". That's the thought. Then you experience fear. That's the emotion. What if you thought "I'm so excited. I'm going to Hawaii?" Your emotion might be joy instead of fear. Do you see how what you think affects how you feel?

Let's try some more:

Antecedent: Your spouse leaves you.
Thought: You think "I'll never find anyone again".
Emotion: You feel depression.

Antecedent: You are driving on freeway and are cut of by another driver.
Thought: You think "He must be in a hurry".
Emotion: You feel sympathy.

Try some of your own. How does the "antecedent, thought, emotion" cycle operate for you?

*Antecedent—Thought—Emotion Cycle*
Antecedent:
Thought:
Emotion:

Antecedent:
Thought:
Emotion:

Antecedent:
Thought:
Emotion:

The reason why thinking can cause negative emotions is that many people engage in twisted thinking. Here is a list of the different forms of twisted thinking. Do you see your thinking patterns in this list?

**Forms of Twisted Thinking:**
- **All or Nothing:** This is black and white thinking with no shades of gray. You are either on or off a diet. One cookie and you think "I've blown it."

- **Overgeneralization:** On the basis of one instance you make a sweeping generalization. You use the words always and never. For example, " I always blow my diets when I eat out."
- **Mental Filter:** You use a mental filter when you focus on only one thing, such as focusing only on the negative. For example, you follow your food plan for six days but only focus on the one day you didn't, and then think " I am such a failure."
- **Discounting the Positive:** When something good happens you ignore or minimize it. You say "no big deal anyone could have done that."
- **Jumping to Conclusions:** You reach a conclusion, usually negative even though there is no evidence to support it. For example, your friend doesn't call you when she said she would and you assume that means she's mad at you.
- **Magnification:** With magnification, negative events are blown out of proportion. Your friends order a pizza and you eat one piece and spend the rest of the day hating yourself for it.
- **Emotional Reasoning:** You misinterpret an event because of the emotional state you are in.
- **Should Statements:** "Shoulds" are unreasonable absolutes that have no place in your life! Preferences are better!
- **Labeling:** You attach a label, such as lazy or stupid to yourself because of a single event or behavior.
- **Personalization and Blame:** Personalization occurs when you accept responsibility for something that you have no control over. For example, you hate yourself for having large hips. Blame occurs when you attribute fault to someone else. For example, you blame your husband for your weight gain because he refuses to go on a diet with you.
- **Catastrophizing:** Catastrophizing occurs when you think of the worse case scenario every time anything happens. You expect the worse. It's "What if-ing!"

Stacey was a wizard at using catastrophizing. She recently purchased her first home and within minutes of moving in her mind was off and running, "What if I lose my job and can't pay the mortgage? What if the roof leaks? What if I hate it here? What if I meet someone and want to get married? What if, what if, what if...." Are you a "what if-er?"

Using the examples you cited above in the last exercise, untwist your thinking and see if you can create a different emotional experience.

### More Logical Thinking

Antecedent:

New thought:

New Emotion:


Antecedent:

New Thought:

New Emotion:


Antecedent:

New Thought:

New Emotion:

Wow! You've learned a lot this week! How's your thinking now? Are you noticing how your thoughts affect your emotions? And how your emotions affect your eating? I hope so! When you are ready, let's continue.

# Week Nine:

## Discovering Your True Hungers ~ Recognizing WHEN You Overeat

Week Nine: Discovering Your True Hungers ~Recognizing When You Overeat

### Am I Really Hungry?

You may recall that at the end of Week Six I gave you a glimpse of what was to come. I addressed the question " How do you stop overeating?" I answered the question by telling you that getting in touch with yourself and your true hunger is the way. In this week and the three that follow you will be learning to identify your true hungers- both physical and psychological. We will start with physical hunger.

The first thing to do when you start eating is to ask yourself "Am I really hungry?" Is there a physical need presenting itself? Unfortunately for many people struggling with emotional overeating, the answer is usually "I don't know." If you don't know if you are physically hungry, you probably are not.

To get in touch with your physical hunger you need to learn the signs and symptoms of hunger. What does physical hunger feel like to you? There are many physical signs of hunger. Some are: grumbling or gurgling noises in the stomach; a feeling of lightheadedness or dizziness; a headache; feeling spacey; or, having trouble concentrating. What are your physical signs of hunger? Do you know? If you don't know, allow yourself to get hungry and check it out.

*My Physical Signs of Hunger Are:*

_____

_____

_____

_____

_____

_____

_____

_____

_____

_____

Maybe you don't know what your physical signs are. That's okay. After so many years of dieting it is not surprising that you don't know. Give yourself permission to feel hungry during the day and then notice what hunger feels like. In time you will be able to recognize the telltale signs. Then you can fill in the list above.

It is important once you are able to identify your physical hunger that you address it. If you are hungry eat! So many dieters don't let themselves eat when they are hungry. You may find yourself falling into that trap. Or you may find that you try to squelch your hunger with things like coffee, diet soda or raw vegetables. It is important to feed your hunger when it arises for four very important reasons. First, your body is telling you something. It needs food to continue functioning and unless fed it won't be able to operate at maximum capacity. Second, feeding your body when you are hungry helps you distinguish between true physical hunger and psychological hunger. The better you become at this skill the less extra food you will eat and the more weight you will lose. Third, feeding yourself when you are hungry is a way of taking care of yourself. The better you become at feeding yourself when you are hungry the better you will become at feeding yourself in other ways when other needs surface. Fourth, being too hungry is a surefire way to trigger a binge.

This week's assignment is a Hungry Inventory. As with the other Inventories, you will be keeping a record of when you eat, what you eat and how hungry you are when you eat it. You will find your Hunger Inventory in the workbook. Once again, after you have completed it, return here for your assessment.

Your Hunger Inventory gave you a hunger scale to use. We will now take a look at what hunger levels you tend to eat.

### My Hunger Assessment
For each Hunger Scale level, record the number of times you ate.

0: _____
1: _____
2: _____
3: _____
4: _____
5: _____
6: _____
7: _____
8: _____
9: _____
10: _____

At what level do you eat most? A healthy hunger level is around a 7 or 8. If you eat sooner than that you are probably not hungry and are eating for emotional reasons. If you eat later than that you may be too hungry and make poor food choices. What did you learn? Write your observations here.

### *My Hunger Observations*

_____

_____

_____

_____

_____

_____

_____

_____

If you noticed that you tend to eat outside of your physical hunger you may benefit from developing a skill I call "Structured Time." This skill allows you to plan your day so that it is filled with interesting hobbies and activities. When your life is full the tendency to eat outside of hunger diminishes. Take a look at the time of day when you tend to eat outside of hunger and see if you can fill that time in other ways. Here are some ideas:

- If you overeat in the mornings, try catching up on phone calls or take a yoga class.
- If your problem is in the late afternoon try a nap or go to the gym.
- If evenings are your downfall, practice relaxation techniques or take up a new hobby.
- If your tendency is to wake up in the middle of night, you may need a sleep hygiene program to help facilitate a better night's sleep.

Lily was able to really get a handle on her afternoon eating by using the Structured Time skill. Lily noticed that every afternoon around 4pm she would go to the refrigerator and start nibbling. She would nibble all the way to dinner. When she analyzed it, Lily discovered she ate because she was bored. She had always wanted to learn to knit and with a new grandchild on the way now was the perfect time to start. She called a local knitting shop and arranged to have knitting lessons at 4pm twice a week. The other days she would do her "homework" from 4pm until dinner. Lily filled in her afternoon with an activity she enjoyed and healed her boredom and emotional overeating in the process.

What "Structured Time" activities could help you? List them here.

### My Structured Time Ideas

_____

_____

_____

_____

_____

_____

_____

_____

Next we will turn to recognizing where you overeat. Recognizing where you overeat will lead to some interesting discoveries. When you are ready, turn the page.

# WEEK TEN:

## Discovering Your True Hungers ~ Recognizing WHERE You Overeat

Week Ten: Discovering Your True Hungers ~ Recognizing WHERE You Overeat

Beginning this week and for the remainder of the program you will be completing a Recovery Diary. This diary will record all the necessary elements to complete this program. You can find the Recovery Diary in the Workbook.

As for this week, your task is to identify where you overeat. There are many locations where people eat. Some of them are: in the kitchen, in the car, at a restaurant, at a parent or relative's house. In some of these places it is easy to manage what you eat. In others you may find yourself overeating. Using the three inventories you have already completed, identify where you overeat?

*Places Where I Overeat:*

_____

_____

_____

_____

_____

_____

## WHO Do You Really Want?

Identifying where you overeat helps you to recognize WHO you really need. For example, if you always overeat when you are alone in the kitchen maybe you need a trustworthy friend. If you overeat every time you walk into your mother's house, maybe you need a warm nurturing parent. Look over your list. See if you can identify the "missing person" that location represents. Once you do that you will be on your way to finding that person and bringing that person into your life. When he or she is in your life you will feel fuller and your need to overeat will diminish. By identifying WHOM you really need in your life, you can go about bringing them to you. If you tend to eat because you are lonely, this task will take away a lot of your emotional overeating.

*People I Really Need:*

_____

_____

_____

_____

_____

_____

Now that you have identified WHOM you need, you need a plan for bringing them into your life. What can you do to find these people and make them part of your life? Annabelle realized she needed a new best friend when she discovered that she did most of her overeating at brunch. Until her former best friend moved across country because of a job transfer, Annabelle had a steady Sunday brunch buddy. Every Sunday they would meet at a different restaurant and catch up in the events of the week. It was Annabelle's favorite time of the week. Since her friend moved, Annabelle would go to brunch by herself and eat much more than her body required. She was trying to fill the void her absent friend created. Annabelle set out to find a new brunch buddy. She went back to her church and got active again. Within several weeks Annabelle had so many new friends she could barely keep up!

## *My People Plan Of Action*

_____

_____

_____

_____

_____

_____

_____

It is time to learn another skill. Last week, you were introduced to the skill called *Structured Time*. This week you will learn the skill called *Eating Without Distraction*. Did you know that food tastes better when you pay attention to it? Try an experiment. The next time you choose to eat something sit down with it. Close your eyes and take a bite. Pay attention to how it tastes, its texture, and its consistency. What do you notice? Then distract yourself. Turn on the television. Read a book. Do something and then take a bite. Does it taste the same? Do you even notice it? When you take the time to really taste the food you are eating you get more satisfaction from it. When you get more satisfaction from your food, you actually eat less. Over time this skill alone can reduce your weight considerably. Try it out. Record your results below.

## *Taste-Test Results*

_____

_____

_____

_____

_____

_____

_____

_____

_____

_____

_____

Time to move on. Ready. Set. Go!

# WEEK ELEVEN:

## Discovering Your True Hungers
## Recognizing What Foods You Overeat

Week Eleven: Discovering Your True Hungers ~ Recognizing WHAT Foods You Overeat

There are certain foods that overeaters tend to overeat. They include: ice cream, chips and sweets. Interestingly, the food we choose to overeat represent a need that isn't being fulfilled. Just like identifying where we eat helped your learn what people are missing from your life, identifying the foods you overeat helps identify the needs that are not being met.

Here are some examples to help you. Many people overeat ice cream or other soft creamy foods (such as mashed potatoes) when they need comforting. Others overeat chips when they need to express anger. Sweets are a common choice for people who had a "sour" day or who are feeling depressed. Meat is for people who need strength and courage. If you overeat foods that remind you of home or your childhood, you may be lonely or homesick. Spend some time thinking about the foods you overeat and what needs they might represent. We will use your responses in the following section.

*Food I Overeat And The Needs They May Represent:*

_____

_____

_____

_____

_____

_____

_____

## WHAT Do You Really Need?

Understanding your food choices and the underlying needs they represent help you answer the question, "What do you really need?" Once you understand what it is you really need you can do something to get it. Let's take some examples to illustrate. Let's say that you eat mashed potatoes and gravy every time you feel sick. If you think about it you may recall that your mother served you mashed potatoes every time you were sick. You also realize that when you are sick you feel sort of vulnerable and lonely. What you really need is to be taken care of. You are eating the mashed potatoes to feel taken care of. Next time you are sick instead of eating potatoes and gravy, call a friend. Ask her to come over and sit with you or to bring you a magazine or a movie. By doing so you will be meeting your real need to being taken care of and you will avoid all the extra calories the potatoes and gravy would supply. Here's another example. You just got off work and you meet some friends for happy hour. You are really angry and stressed out. It had been a rough week. So, now you are at happy hour and they are offering free salsa and chips. You love chips and you start eating and eating and eating. The crunch sure feels good. Crunching on the chips is relieving your anger. What you really need is to express anger. Eating chips relieves some of the stress associated with anger but doesn't get rid of the anger itself. So what you really need is to get rid of the anger. You can do that talking about it, writing about it, or being assertive with the person with whom you are angry.

Take the needs you identified in the exercise above and see if you can figure out some other ways to meet them. Then the next time they present themselves you will have a choice of how to respond. You can eat or you can do something else.

### *Meeting My Real Needs*

_____

_____

_____

_____

_____

_____

_____

_____

I hope that by now you are really grasping how your feelings affect your eating. The ways you use food to meet your emotional needs are becoming clearer to you. If they are not, review Weeks Ten and Eleven before continuing to Week Twelve. Wendy needed to do just that. This week proved to be particularly difficult for her. She struggled a bit understanding what her real needs are. With my encouragement she spent two more weeks on this material before moving on. Although initially resistant to the idea of staying put, Wendy followed my suggestion and made great headway on identifying her needs. When she was ready she moved on and her progress through the rest of the program never faltered.

# WEEK TWELVE:

## Discovering Your True Hungers ~ Recognizing WHY You Overeat

Week Twelve: Discovering Your True Hungers ~Recognizing WHY You Overeat

Your responses from last week identified some of the needs that your overeating is addressing. This information will be a big help in this week which focuses on the underlying reasons why you overeat.

As I mentioned earlier, you overeat for some very important reasons. Overeating is serving an important purpose for you. Until you identify that purpose your success at weight loss will be short-lived. You must identify the underlying reasons for your overeating and address them in constructive ways or the weight will not stay off. You will continue to overeat despite of your best dieting efforts. Thus, recognizing why you overeat is the focus of this week. We will look at fears, purposes, and feelings.

### What Do You Really FEAR?
There are many, many feelings that cause people to overeat. The most common ones are stress and anxiety. The basis for the stress and anxiety is fear

Fears such as:
+ Fear of intimacy
+ Fear of failure
+ Fear of success

- Fear of being seen
- Fear of being heard
- Fear of not being seen
- Fear of not being heard
- Fear of not being perfect
- Fear of being perfect
- Fear of not being liked
- Fear of not being good enough
- Fear of being too good
- Fear of not being smart enough
- Fear of not being pretty or handsome enough
- Fear of being thin

Overeaters as a group tend to be anxious people. They tend to experience more stress than their non-overeating counterparts. They walk around more frightened and less confident than non-overeaters. Truthfully, there is no reason for this. Overeaters are just as competent, capable, and attractive as other people. They just don't know it! Could this be you?

By overeating you are avoiding dealing with these fears. By avoiding your fears you experience less anxiety. Your overeating is serving you by keeping your anxiety in check. Have you ever noticed yourself actually calming down as you eat? That's anxiety reduction in action. Pay attention the next time you find yourself overeating and see if you feel yourself calming down with each bite of food that goes in your mouth.

### Other Purposes Overeating Serves

Other purposes that overeating (and consequently being overweight) serves include:
- Avoiding relationships
- Avoiding responsibility for one's life

- Being lazy
- Being less than perfect
- Not failing (because you are not really trying)
- Staying safe

Think about why you may be overeating and what purpose it may serve for you. Look over your answers to the previous questions for clues. It may take some time for you to get a clear picture of this. That's okay. Take your time. You can come back to this question and add more to it later as answers surface. For now, do your best and write down what comes to mind. Often it is our first answer that is the "right" one.

### *Reasons Why I Overeat:*

_____
_____
_____
_____
_____
_____
_____
_____

Overeaters are also frightened of feelings. They often eat in response to uncomfortable feelings, both positive and negative. In the next section, we will take a look at a wide range of feelings that trigger overeating and offer solutions for coping with them, instead of turning to food.

### Feeling "THE FEELINGS"

As you know, there are many moods and feelings that can trigger the urge to eat. They include:

- Anger
- Anxiety

- Boredom
- Depression
- Fatigue
- Fear
- Frustration
- Hyperactivity
- Insomnia
- Loneliness
- Physical aches and pains
- Sadness
- Stress

We'll take each one at a time. First, we will address anger.

**Anger:**

Anger is an intense emotion that comes from a belief that you have been unfairly treated. Some physical manifestations of anger include clenched jaw, stiffening body, and thoughts of revenge. For many, anger is an emotion to be feared and avoided. Some people go to great lengths not to express this emotion because they are afraid of it. They are afraid that if they allow their anger to emerge it will overwhelm them. They are afraid of what they might do or say because of their anger. In an effort to avoid angry, many overeaters eat it away. They suppress anger feelings with food.

Anger is not an emotion to be feared. It is an emotion to express. Healthy expression of anger is a vital skill that everyone can learn. Here are some tips to help you express your anger in a way that helps not hurts you:

- Address your anger in the moment it occurs rather than let it fester and grow by holding on to it
- Use assertive language to say what you need to say
- If expressing your anger directly to the person who angered you is not possible or too scary, you can express your anger in other ways, such as, writing about in a journal or unmailed letter, telling a trusted friend or therapist
- Physically express your anger by exercising, running, walking, hitting tennis balls, shooting baskets
- A more creative expression of anger is writing the name of the person or situation that angers you on the sole of your shoe and stomping around
- Write the offending name or situation on a dozen raw eggs and break them against the shower wall
- Cry or yell into a pillow; hit your mattress with a tennis racket
- Using the Anger Letter in the Workbook write out your feelings. Do not send the letter. Use it as a tool to release your feelings.

Anxiety:

Anxiety is fear of the future. It is the apprehension of unpleasant or dangerous events. It is the thoughts that you tell yourself in response to a particular situation or occurrence. It is the way you explain things to yourself. Anxiety is, in a way, "all in your head!" even though it feels like it is all in your body. The physical symptoms of anxiety are quite real— sweaty palms, dizziness, headaches, heart palpitations, lightheadedness. But the truth is you create your own anxiety by the way you talk you yourself. This is actually good news. Because if you can talk yourself into anxiety you can talk yourself out of it. For example, let's say you are going on a job interview and you are understandably nervous. But as you are driving to the interview you start getting really nervous. Why? What's going on that has you getting more anxious? Is it something you are thinking about as you drive to your interview? Your conversation with yourself probably goes something like this:

*"I gotta get this job. If I don't get this job I don't know what I'll do. I only have a little bit of money left in my savings account. What will I do if I don't get this job? How will I pay the rent? Where will I live if I can't afford my apartment anymore? Where will I go? I'll end up on the street. How will I survive? What will I do? There is a donut shop. I want one NOW! I need one if I am going to survive this day!"*

By now you are a wreck and on your way to a binge. You've gone from simple normal nervousness over a job interview to being homeless and living on the streets. Sound absurd? Well, unfortunately this kind of self-talk is quite common.

What would a more healthful, supportive inner dialogue sound like? How about something like this:

*"Boy am I nervous. I really want this job. I know I have the qualifications but the competition is stiff. I really hope I get this job. But if I don't I know I'll be okay. I still have some money left in my savings account, so I won't be on the streets! I will continue to look for work. I'll send out more resumes. Oh! I know I'll call Susan. She'll have some good ideas for my job search. In the meanwhile I'll give this interview my best shot and go from there."*

This second conversation is much more supportive and constructive. It builds you up and gives you hope rather than tear you down and make you want to binge. It is this kind of positive self-talk that alleviates anxiety, builds self-esteem, and reduces the urge to binge.

Thus, the first step to dealing with anxiety is to "treat" your thoughts. To change how you explain things to yourself so that you see things in a more positive way. To say things to yourself such as "everything will be okay" or "all I am experiencing is anxiety- it can't hurt me." Once you get used to talking to yourself in this more positive way much of your anxiety will disappear.

Another way to deal with anxiety is to practice relaxation techniques. One to try is a systematic muscle relaxing journey. With a gentle, calm and reassuring voice read the following into a tape recorder and then lie back in a darkened room and enjoy yourself as you relax.

*"Close your eyes. Lie back on a sofa or floor and just relax. Pay attention to your breathing. Listen to your breaths as they float in and out, in and out. Allow the thoughts from the day to pass gently through your mind. In and out. Count to yourself, slowly, from one to ten. Relaxing deeply with each count. Ready? One, two, three, four, five, six, seven, eight, nine, and ten. Now starting with your feet relax each part of your body. Begin by tightly clenching your toes for a count of ten (one, two, three, four, five, six, seven, eight, nine, ten.) Now release. Feel the tingling as your feet let go of the tensions of the day. Let's repeat your feet. Again, clench your toes for a count of ten (one, two, three, four, five, six, seven, eight, nine, ten.) Now release. Doesn't that feel good. Now move up to your calves. Tighten your calves for the count of ten and then release. Ready? Tighten (one, two, three, four, five, six, seven, eight, nine, ten.) Release. Feel the relaxation move up your body from your feet through your calves. Let's repeat your calves. Ready? Tighten (one, two, three, four, five, six, seven, eight, nine, ten.) Release. Allow the relaxation to fill up your body. Breathe deeply. In and out. In and out. Feel yourself becoming more and more relaxed with each breath. Allow yourself to relax a bit more and then continue with your thighs. Tighten your thighs for a count of ten (one, two, three, four, five, six, seven, eight, nine, ten.) Release. Allow the relaxation to move further up your body. Enjoy the tingling. Enjoy the breathing. If a thought pops into your mind gently push it out. There will be plenty of time to think about it later, after your relaxation is complete. For now, just relax and truly enjoy this time you are giving yourself. When you are ready move on to your arms.*

*Clench your fists and tighten your arms as hard as you can. Hold for a count of ten (one, two, three, four, five, six, seven, eight, nine, ten) and release. Let the relaxation float up your arms. Continue to relax your legs. You should be feeling pretty good by now. Continue to breath. In and out. In and out. Now relax your shoulders. As hard as you can squeeze your shoulder blades together for a count of ten (one, two, three, four, five, six, seven, eight, nine, ten.) Release. Shrug them up and down a few times to get more kinks out. Now repeat your arms and then your shoulders. Clench your fists and arms for a count of ten (one, two, three, four, five, six, seven, eight, nine, ten.)Release. Feel yourself sink further and further into the surface on which you are lying. Now, squeeze your shoulder blades together as hard as you can. Hold for ten (one, two, three, four, five, six, seven, eight, nine, ten.)Release. Feels good. Breathe in and out. In and out. Allow your body to sink further into the surface on which you are lying. Relax. Just relax. Now for your face. Scrunch your face as hard as you can. Don't worry no one is watching! You are alone relaxing. Scrunch for a count of ten (one, two, three, four, five, six, seven, eight, nine, ten.) Release. Can you feel the tension leaving your face? Let's do your face again. Ready? Scrunch for ten (one, two, three, four, five, six, seven, eight, nine, ten.) Release. Relax. Relax deeply and serenely. Allow yourself to enjoy the floating sensation that is welling inside of you. Enjoy the quiet. Enjoy the tranquillity. If there is any part of your body that is still feeling tense, isolate it and then tighten and release. Tighten and release. Now continue to relax. Let the thoughts float in and out of your mind. Let the peacefulness take over and just relax. Lie here for a few minutes and enjoy the rest. When you are ready count gently from ten down to one and open your eyes (ten, nine, eight, seven, six, five, four, three, two, one.) Open your eyes. You feel relaxed and ready to take on life! Go for it!*

In addition to using the relaxation exercise that you just learned, there are two other ways for you to reduce the anxiety in your life. They are:

- Physical activity: Running, walking, swimming, gardening are all helpful in reducing anxiety because they expend energy. Anxiety can be thought of as an energy buzzing through you. If you expend some of that energy through physical exercise less will "buzz" and you will feel better.
- Eliminate caffeine. For many people the side effects of caffeine mimic anxiety. They are racing heart, sweaty palms, nervous stomach, and sleepless nights. If you suffer from any of these conditions you may want to eliminate caffeine and see if you feel calmer. Check labels. There is caffeine in some items you might never think about such as headache medicine and tea.

Now that you have some ways to deal with anxiety, we will move on to Boredom.

### Boredom:

Boredom is either a lack of interesting activities or being prevented from doing something interesting. If you are feeling under stimulated, restless, with empty time on your hands, you may be feeling bored. To cope with this feeling, it is important to add interests, activities and relationships to your life. Here are some ideas to get you started.

- Call a friend and go to the movies
- Make new friends by joining a sports team or charitable organization
- Try a new hobby
- Take a class to your local adult education program
- Try a new sport
- Read the latest best-seller
- Exercise
- Learn a new language (how about sign?)
- Call into a talk radio show
- Knit a sweater
- Make homemade gifts

There is another aspect to boredom that needs to be addressed. For some people, boredom is actually an indirect expression of anger. Check that out for yourself. Are you feel angry about something but cannot express it? Are you withdrawing and isolating and as a result feeling bored because of unexpressed anger? If you are review the section above on anger and see if you can find a way to release your angry feelings. If you can, I suspect your feelings of boredom will go away.

### Depression:

The next feeling we will tackle is depression. Depression comes in several forms. It can feel like the blues. A general sort of blah feeling when you are just not yourself. It can come in the form of anxiety and agitation when you find yourself irritable with everyone and everything around you. It can also be more serious when you find yourself unable to accomplish even the most basic things in your life, such as getting up to go to work or showering when you get dressed in the morning. You may feel tired, in pain or "prickly." You may experience changes in your sleeping and eating patterns, as well. Sometimes your concentration disappears as does interest in things you used to enjoy. If your depression so severe that it significantly impacts your life I urge you to get professional assistance to deal with it. A good psychotherapist and perhaps some medication can do wonders for a severe depression. See your physician for a referral or call your local chapter of the American Psychological Association for assistance.

For the less serious forms of depression there is quite a bit you can do for yourself to cope. The first step is to identify why you are feeling depressed. Have you suffered a loss lately? Did someone criticize you and you are feeling badly now? Are you disappointed about something? Are you angry about something? Once you have identified the source of your depression, describe it. Write about, talk about, draw about. Any expression of it is helpful. Then take action. Action is an effective antidote for depression. Do something. Go for a walk. Make a phone call. Read a book. Paint a picture. Anything. Get moving. Just take action.

### Fatigue:

Most people don't think of fatigue as a feeling but it is. And it is one that leads to a lot of overeating. If you overeat because you are tired, you would do better to address your fatigue with something more likely to rest and restore you than food. Here are some ideas.

+ Take a nap
+ Go for a walk
+ Meditate
+ Use a relaxation technique like the one described above

### Fear:

Fear is a physical "alarm" or warning of danger. It can feel like anxiety, so use the techniques discussed above in the anxiety section to help you with your fears.

### Frustration:

To cope with frustration identify the source of your frustration and confront it. State your wishes, needs, and desires clearly and assertively. Too much frustration can lead to anger, so I encourage you to manage your frustration in a timely fashion.

### Hyperactivity:

Hyperactivity means that you keep yourself busy with lots and lots of obligations, tasks and activities. For some people doing so is a way to avoid issues and problems they don't want to deal with. To end hyperactivity you need to figure out what it is you are trying to avoid and address it. Usually there is some uncomfortable underlying feeling that is being avoided. If that is true for you the best course of action is feeling the feeling and dealing with the problem directly either on your own or in therapy.

Insomnia:

Do you have trouble falling asleep? Or staying asleep throughout the night? If so you may suffer from insomnia. To cope with insomnia see your physician to rule out any medical reasons for your sleeplessness. Then adopt some simple techniques to help you get a better night's sleep. These techniques are often referred to as "sleep hygiene." For example:

- End your day with some relaxation techniques, a warm bath or warm milk.
- Use your bedroom for sleep and sex only.
- Leave your work life outside your bedroom.
- Turn the TV off. Watch the news in the morning instead of the evening to create a calmer sense of well-being at night.

Loneliness:

When you are lonely you experience distress from the absence of inter-personal relationships. If loneliness is the reason you overeat, try some of the following suggestions to add more people into your life.

- Join a church or synagogue and attend regularly
- Take a class
- Volunteer for a cause you believe in
- Get a dog or cat
- Offer to baby sit a neighbor's children
- Spend time with your family
- Contact old friends you haven't heard from in a while
- Join a support group to build relationship skills

Sometimes a person can heal her pain from loneliness by developing a healthier relationship with herself. In the Workbook, you will find a template for a letter to yourself. It is called " Love Myself Letter". The next time you are feeling lonely, write yourself a letter. See if that helps you feel better.

**Physical Aches and Pains:**
Physical discomfort causes some people to eat. This behavior usually started in childhood when a child was offered a treat after skinning her knee. She learned to associate physical pain with food and a lifelong habit began. To end this habit, deal with your physical pain directly.

- See a doctor, chiropractor or physical therapist
- Get a massage
- Take a bath
- Soak in a Jacuzzi
- Exercise
- Get some rest
- Take time off to recuperate

**Sadness:**
Sadness is that unhappy feeling you experience when you lose something or someone and is usually experienced as tears, withdrawal, and a slumped body posture. Unaddressed, sadness could lead to depression. To cope with sadness, acknowledge your loss. Grieve it. Allow yourself to have your feelings. They will soon pass and you will feel happy again.

**Stress:**
People probably do more eating in response to stress than to anything else. To overcome overeating it is imperative that you learn others ways to cope with stress. Participating in regular stress-reducing activities is a good way to do just that. Here are some ideas to get you started:

- Meditate
- Exercise
- Stretch
- Get massages
- Listen to soothing music
- Read
- Practice relaxation techniques

- Deep breathing
- Stroke a pet
- Cradle a sleeping child
- Sip some herbal tea
- Turn off your phone and pager

We will cover even more ways to cope with your feelings without overeating later on.

### *"Drop and Give Me Ten"*

It takes time to identify your feelings. In the beginning you may identify them after the fact. That is after the binge. Here's why. When you are in a binge you are anxious. As the food takes effect, you calm down. When you calm down you can think straight. When you think straight you can figure out what happened and what you were feeling. Later as you get better at identifying your reasons for overeating and identifying your feelings you will be able to do so during the binge. Then when you get really good at identifying your feelings, you will identify them before the binge. At that point you will be able to choose what you want to do. You may choose to eat. That's okay. At least you will know what you are doing and why you are doing it. You will have a choice and that will give you control over your eating. Until you get to that point you may want to practice a technique I call *"Drop and Give Me Ten."* During a binge, sit down. Wherever you are just sit. It doesn't matter if it's in the kitchen in front of an open refrigerator door. Just sit. That's the "Drop" part. While you are sitting don't eat. Instead count to ten. You can count aloud or silently. It doesn't matter how you count, just count. Take a deep breath at ten and then continue eating if you still want to. If not, put the food back and continue what you were doing before the binge began. This technique of *"Drop and Give Me Ten"* is an excellent way to regain some control over your eating when you feel you lose it during a binge. Many of my patients say they are able to stop a binge with this technique. Others say it helps them get in touch with their feelings. You try it. See what it does for you.

This has been a very full week with lots of new and exciting information. Take a few moments to reflect on what you've learned so far. Summarize your main points below.

*My Points From Week Twelve*

_____

_____

_____

_____

_____

_____

_____

_____

### Rediscover your True Hungers

You've come a long way since you started. You can feel quite proud of yourself. You have accomplished a lot. This week we began putting everything you have learned so far together. To review, you have learned that to end overeating for good you must discover your true hungers. Your physical hunger and your emotional hunger. Physical hunger is the hunger that you satisfy with food and drink. It is the hunger that keeps your body fueled and operating at maximum efficiency. Emotional hunger is the hunger that you try to satisfy with food because that is your habit but that remains after you have eaten because emotional hunger is not about food. Emotional hunger is about feelings. It is about understanding and addressing your underlying needs and desires. It means crying when you are sad. It means smiling when you are feeling happy. It means expressing anger when you are feeling vexed.

To rediscover your true hungers you need to take time before you eat to ask yourself "What am I really hungry for?" If the answer is food, you eat. If the answer is a hug, a bath, or a nap, you provide yourself with those necessities.

Now it's time for you to review what you have learned about yourself and your need so far. Pulling from your answers to previous exercises, see if you can answer the question, "What Am I Truly Hungry For?"

### *I Am Truly Hungry For:*

_____

_____

_____

_____

_____

_____

_____

_____

and the question, "What Can I Do To Meet My True Hungers?"

### *I Can Meet My True Hungers By:*

_____

_____

_____

_____

_____

_____

_____

_____

**Becoming The Person You Want To Be**

The bonus in committing yourself to this process of overcoming overeating is that you bring out the best in you. Through the work you are doing you are learning more about yourself and your behavior than you ever have before. As a result you have the chance to become the person you always wanted to be. Who is that person? Describe your "ideal self" here.

*My Ideal Self*

_____

_____

_____

_____

_____

_____

_____

_____

Are you close to your ideal self? If not what do you need to do to get there?

_____

_____

_____

_____

_____

_____

_____

You can also use a tool I call "Photojournalism" to help you become your "ideal self." In the Workbook are instructions for creating an "Image Page." In essence, an Image Page is a collage of pictures that depict what you would like your life to be about. It's a fun project and one you can do with others. I had one patient, Abbey, who set up an image page party. She invited several friends to get together. She asked them each to bring several magazines and they spent hours together creating their life visions.

### Build Better Relationships

Another bonus is that you will also build the skills to have better relationships. Relationships are tricky things. If you have suffered from overeating for any significant amount of time chances are your relationships have suffered too. Perhaps you find yourself in an unhappy relationship and you have been using food as a way to avoid leaving. Or maybe you are not in a relationship and the reason is because you have been using your food as a way to isolate and avoid relationships. Maybe you are a sneak eater and in doing that you are keeping secrets in your relationships. How has your relationship with food influenced your relationships with people? Think about it for a while and record your thoughts here.

*My Relationships*

_____

_____

_____

_____

_____

_____

_____

It is now time to move on to learn other ways to deal with the problems and situations in your life. In Week Thirteen, you will learn new ways to cope.

# WEEK THIRTEEN:

## Learning New Ways To Cope

Week Thirteen: Learning New Ways to Cope

In order to overcome overeating, it is vital to make your life about more than food. You may have spent so much time, energy, and money on diets and binges that your life has lost its balance. In learning how to live your life without turning to excess food, you will be learning new ways to cope with your life. Once we take food, diets, and bingeing out of your repertoire of activities to occupy yourself with you will need to find other things to fill up your time and your life. These new activities will provide a much needed break for those inevitable stressful times. Your first task is to find something else to do that interests you, for example, find a hobby, get a job, volunteer, join a book club, go back to school, take art classes, learn to dance, or train for a marathon. Have an outlet, an interest, so that when times get rough and you need a break you have another "release valve" instead of the refrigerator.

The next task in your quest to be free from overeating is learning to deal with underlying emotions. Such as, learning to express and appreciate anger or to feel sad when you are sad or to let anxiety fill you up so it will pass. Using positive self-talk and writing in a journal are other examples. Now that you have the general idea, let's get specific.

## When You Need a Break

If most of your overeating occurs when you are stressed, over-whelmed or tired, chances are you need a break! Learning how to build refreshing and rejuvenating breaks into your daily schedule is an excellent way to overcome stress and fatigue eating. One idea is to make exercise a part of your life. Another is to practice relaxation techniques and yoga. Or you can find an interesting hobby.

## When You Need to Cry

If your overeating is in response to uncomfortable emotions, the way to cope is to learn to feel those emotions. We spoke earlier of allowing yourself to have your feelings. If you need to cry, cry. If you need to pout, pout.

## When You Need to Scream

If your overeating is an expression of anger, you need to allow yourself to be angry. In a previous week we reviewed several ways for you to express your anger. Take some time to look at them again and start practicing the ones that feel acceptable to you. Once you "find your voice" and can express your anger, you will see a real reduction in the amount of binge eating you do.

## When You Need to Feel Better About Yourself

Most of the time the reason a person feels badly about herself is because of the things she tells herself about who she is and the life she leads. This "self-talk" is usually negative. A key to improving your relationship with yourself and feeling better about who you are is learning to change negative self-talk into positive self-talk. The trick to making such a change is becoming aware of the negative self-talk you engage in. For the next few days start to pay attention to what you tell yourself. Listen for how you explain things to yourself. Are you explaining them in a positive way or a negative way? Is your glass half-full or half-empty? Do you have enough of something or do you need much more? Use the space provided to records your thoughts.

### *My Negative Script*

_____

_____

_____

_____

_____

_____

_____

Once you have noticed how much negative self-talk you engage in, the next step is to rephrase those negative thoughts into positive ones. Your positive thoughts need to be believable and realistic for this process to be successful. Here's an example. Let's say you said the following negative thought to yourself "I'm hopeless. I'll never get this right. I'll always overeat." To change that negative monologue into a positive one try something like this "I have struggled in the past to overcome overeating. I am now trying again and this time I will give it my all and enjoy the small changes I make along the way." Thoughts like that one are encouraging and supportive. Statements like the ones I suggest are more constructive than to say "I'll never eat chocolate again!" A statement like that one is a set up for failure and more self-defeating talk.

Using your negative script from above, rephrase your thoughts into more positive ones. I have given you some space to do that.

### *My Positive Self-Talk*

_____

_____

_____

_____

_____

_____

_____

## When You Need to Change Your Life

If you are feeling as if your entire life is not working, then it is time for some goal setting. Goal setting is an effective way to make serious changes in your life. For goal setting to be effective you must write down your goals. And your goals must be concrete, realistic, and attainable. To set a goal that you want to weigh 100 pounds when you are 5'10" is unrealistic and unattainable. A goal of 150 pounds is more likely. You can set goals for any area of your life that you would like to improve. Using the formula I describe below you can achieve anything you set your mind to.

### *Goal Setting*

1. Write down what you want to achieve in your life. Here are some areas to consider:
   - work/career
   - health
   - money
   - love/relationships
   - education
   - lifestyle
   - travel
   - leisure
   - personal growth

_____

_____

_____

_____

_____

_____

2. Looking at what you have written in step one, create goals you can achieve in 5 years. Write them in the affirmative as if they have already been achieved. For example, "In 5 years, I am living in a condominium with a swimming pool."

_____

_____

_____

_____

_____

_____

_____

_____

3. Now take your five year goals and divide them into one year goals. Write your one year goals in the affirmative as well. For example, "By the end of this year I will have saved $1,000 towards the down payment for my condominium."

_____

_____

_____

_____

_____

_____
_____
_____

4. Do the same thing for 6 month goals.

_____
_____
_____
_____
_____
_____
_____
_____
_____

5. Now for 1 month goals.

_____
_____
_____
_____
_____
_____
_____
_____

6. And, 1 week goals. For example, "This week I will open a savings account for my down payment."

_____
_____
_____
_____
_____

_____

_____

7. Once you have your weekly goals prepared you can assign daily tasks. Try to do one or two tasks each day towards your goals and before long you will be well on your way to achieving them.

_____

_____

_____

_____

_____

_____

_____

_____

_____

8. Remember to review your goals on a regularly basis. How often will you review your goals? Write your commitment here. "I will review my goals every _____ days/ weeks/ months."

In addition to the exercises you just did, there is a Goal Setting Worksheet in Part Four and two additional techniques below to help you achieve your goals.

### *Creative Visualization*

Creative Visualization is a technique that encourages you to use your imagination to see in your "mind's eye" your goal achieved. It is a form of daydreaming except that it is deliberate and focused. To use Creative Visualization to help you achieve your goals, follow the steps outlined here.

Step 1. Decide on a goal which you would like to achieve. Let's take the condominium with the swimming pool as an example.

Step 2. Lie down or sit in a comfortable chair and close your eyes.

Step 3. With your eyes closed allow your body to relax and your mind to quite down. Then when you are relaxed, create an image or picture in your mind of your goal. Imagine it with lots of detail. See yourself in it. For example, see yourself in the swimming pool of your new condominium. Or, imagine yourself furnishing the condo and having a cup of tea at your kitchen table. Allow the image to unfold. Enjoy yourself. This activity can be a lot of fun. Think of your goal in present tense as if it already exists. Continue to picture yourself with it or in it now.

Step 4. When you are ready slowly open your eyes but hold the image with you for a few seconds.

Step 5. Focus on your image often. For example, when you are standing in line at the bank or sitting in a waiting room for your dentist appointment to start. Think about your image in a positive exciting way.

Step 6. Repeat this exercise daily until your goal is achieved.

### The Pink Balloon
The Pink Balloon technique is an off-shoot of the Creative Visualization technique. Follow these simple steps daily to help bring a goal to life.

Step 1. Start in a relaxed position either sitting or lying down with your eyes closed.

Step 2. Imagine your goal in as much detail as you can. Hold the image in your "mind's eye" for a minute or two. Really let it come into focus.

Step 3. Using your imagination, surround your goal with a pink balloon.

Step 4. Now in your mind, let go of balloon and imagine it loating in the universe attracting and gathering energy for your goal's manifestation.

Step 5. When you are ready, open your eyes knowing that you are making your goal happen.

## Ineffective Coping Skills

This week's focus is on learning new ways to cope with the problems in your life. Here is a list of "ineffective" coping skills. I call them "ineffective" because in my opinion they do not correct the problems you face. Instead, they serve to distract you and turn your time and energy away from the real issues. Yet these are the coping "skills" that many people use to manage their lives. Take a look at the list. Do you do any of them? If so, see if you can replace these ineffective coping skills with the effective ones on the next list.

- Eating
- Smoking
- Drinking
- Taking recreational drugs
- Abusing prescription drugs
- Trying to forget about the whole thing

- Wishing it will go away
- Taking your feelings out on others
- Distracting yourself
- Fantasizing
- Leaving it to fate
- Isolating/withdrawing
- Resigning yourself that nothing can be done
- Criticizing yourself
- Hoping for a miracle
- Sleeping too much
- Expecting the worst possible outcome
- Denying the problem
- Losing hope that things will ever change
- Overworking
- Pretending nothing happened
- Keeping feelings to yourself
- Entering into destructive relationships

## Effective Coping Skills

Here is a list of "effective" coping skills. Mastering these skills will make your life more successful and pleasurable. Which of these effective coping skills can you learn to use? Try some of them and see which ones feel good to you.

- Stand your ground and fight for what you want
- Express anger to the person who caused the problem
- Let feelings out
- Take a chance and do something risky
- Talk to someone
- Ask someone you respect for advice
- Accept sympathy and understanding from someone

- Get professional help (lawyer, accountant, doctor, therapist)
- If you know what has to be done, do it!
- Make a plan of action and follow through
- Just concentrate on the next step
- Draw on past experiences to get courage and confidence
- Brain storm to come up with different solutions -even outrageous ones
- Talk to yourself to make yourself feel better
- Step back from the situation and be more objective
- Remind yourself of how things could be worse; gain perspective
- Use cognitive rehearsal which means going over in your mind what has to be said or done
- Try to see the positive side of the situation
- Tell yourself that things will get better
- Pray
- Try to learn more about the situation
- Take things one day/step at a time
- Think about how a role model would do it

Which of these effective, healthy coping skills will you try the next time you feel like eating in response to a situation?

*Coping Skills I Will Try:*

_____

_____

_____

_____

_____

_____

In the Workbook, you will find a page called "Other Strategies". Use that sheet to list coping techniques you can employ to make your life run smoother. Here's one you can consider. It was told to me my patient Hannah. When Hannah is angry at someone she gets a carton of eggs. She writes the offending person's name on each of the eggs and gets into the shower. She then throws the eggs one at a time against the shower wall. When she's done she washes the eggs down the drain and says she feels much better!

The ideas, techniques, and suggestion presented in this week are "self-help" measures. They are things you can do on your own to help yourself. Sometimes, however, it is advisable, even necessary, to get professional help. Part Three discusses when it is time to see a professional.

# WEEK FOURTEEN:

## Relapse Prevention

### Week Fourteen: Relapse Prevention Plan

You are almost there. You've almost made it to the end of this program. Your relationship with food, your emotions, and your self should be much improved by now. Congratulations! Good work!

This week we will focus on relapse prevention. By the end of the week you will have a Plan of Action in place to help you through more difficult times. Let's begin with some definitions. A *lapse* is a slip in behavior. It is somewhat predictable and certainly not a major tragedy. It is merely a backslide that can be corrected. The best way to deal with a lapse is to address it immediately. The sooner you recognize a lapse and change your behavior the quicker you will be back on track. If you don't address a lapse quickly, it could lead to a *relapse*. A relapse occurs when you revert back to your "baseline behavior." In other words, your old behaviors become the norm again. To regain your recovery you have to start all over.

By preparing a written plan for anticipated problems you can avoid many lapses and thus avoid the risk of a relapse. This strategy worked well for Sharon. Sharon and her husband were planning a second honeymoon on a cruise. This particular cruise ship was known for its midnight buffets. In the past most of Sharon's emotional overeating occurred at night after her husband went to sleep. She would sneak into the kitchen and raid the refrigerator. A midnight buffet had the potential for being a real set-up for Sharon. So, she planned ahead and wrote a written plan of action for dealing with the buffet. Among the items on her strategy plan were (1) rewarding herself with a piece of jewelry for getting through the cruise without eating at the buffet; (2) asking her husband for help; (3) eating a healthy dinner so she wouldn't be hungry at midnight; and, (4) making love with her husband at midnight instead of eating!

To prepare your Plan of Action, let's take a look at some obstacles you may encounter along the way:

- Holidays can present problems because of all the inviting and delicious foods that are available.
- Social pressure occurs when well-meaning coworkers, siblings, partners, parents, and friends encourage you to eat.
- Vacations, especially cruises and all-inclusive resorts, offer challenges. Particularly when you use a vacation as an excuse to overeat.
- Life changes cause stress and stress can lead to overeating. Events such as a move, a divorce, or a basic change in your routine could lead to excess eating.
- The stress and disruption that illness causes whether your illness or someone else's can be an obstacle to healthy eating habits.
- Hitting a plateau and getting discouraged when you are feeling like you are not making any progress can also thwart your efforts.

Each of these life situations presents risk to your eating behavior. By anticipating these risks and designing a course of action to deal with them you can head them off and keep on track.

Think about the obstacles just presented. Can you anticipate any of them interrupting your progress and success? Are there other obstacles that you can anticipate that were not listed above? Make your list here.

*Obstacles I Need to Prepare For:*

_____

_____

_____

_____

_____

_____

_____

In Part Four, you will find a Plan of Action Worksheet. Use it to create a plan for handling the obstacles you may face. Remember to anticipate obstacles as you go through your life and plan for them wisely. Doing so will keep your emotional and physical health in good form. Use this week to create plans of action for any obstacles you may encounter. Being prepared is your best relapse prevention skill.

You are almost done. When you are ready go on to Week 15.

# WEEK FIFTEEN:

## Putting It All Together Forever

Week Fifteen: Putting it All Together

Well you made it! You have arrived. It's Week Fifteen and you are well on your way to overcoming emotional overeating. I know that this journey has been difficult at times, but you persevered and your rewards are abundant.

By working your way through this program, doing the written exercises, and focusing on your recovery, you probably feel different now. I have listed 30 ways my patients have described the improvements they have felt. Are any of them true for you too?

### 30 Indicators of Recovery:
- Your self-esteem is much improved.
- You see yourself as valuable from the inside rather than the outside.
- You validate your own feelings without judgment.
- You experience unconditional love and acceptance.
- You accept imperfection in yourself and others.
- Your expectations of yourself and others are realistic.
- You have established a support network of professionals, friends, and family.
- You have taken responsibility for yourself and your life.
- You have clarified your own belief system.
- You have learned to protect yourself from abusive situations.

- You have stopped denying the truths about yourself and your eating behavior.
- You have let go of guilt.
- You are leading a balanced life.
- You have established boundaries for yourself and with others.
- You have worked through your issues of loss and grief.
- You can laugh at yourself and your problems.
- You have a realistic view of your body and weight.
- You no longer fear fat or weight.
- You now play an emotionally healthier role with the people in your life.
- You have released the past.
- You live in the present.
- You plan for the future rather than fear it.
- You set emotionally healthy limits for yourself and others.
- You know how to recognize and express feelings.
- You are able to build and maintain intimate relationships.
- You have good communication skills.
- You express yourself well to others.
- You are capable of building trusting relationships.
- You resolve conflict in healthy ways.
- You are your own best friend.

So, how did you do? Are you experiencing any of these recovery indicators? I sincerely hope so. Since you have gotten so good at completing exercises, how about writing about your recovery? As usual, I have provided space for you to do just that!

*My Recovery*

_____

_____

_____

_____

_____

_____

My patients have also come up with 45 Tips for Success. Are you doing any of them? Do you have any of your own to add?

### 45 Tips For Success:

- Always feel your feeling.
- Always say what you mean.
- Plan activities that you enjoy.
- Don't make phone calls from the kitchen!
- For routine trips like going shopping or to work, find a route that does not pass bakeries, fast food restaurants and the like.
- Do boring chores in a food-free zone.
- In situations where you would be tempted to eat (watching TV for example) chew gum or do something with your hands.
- Prepare a shopping list and stick to it.
- Avoid impulse shopping.
- Don't shop on an empty stomach.
- When shopping stick to the perimeter of the store; that's where the healthy foods are.
- Don't go food shopping with the kids.
- Let others buy and store their own snacks.
- Buy snacks in single serving sizes.
- Keep problematic foods out of the house. If it's not in the house you can't eat it!
- Plan treats so you can really enjoy them.
- Keep all food in the kitchen only.
- Serve all food from the kitchen only.
- Store challenging foods in opaque containers.

- Make healthy snacks easy to see and get to.
- Use your Food Awareness Inventory regularly.
- Chew gum while you cook.
- Ask others to help with food preparation.
- If you cook in large quantities, freeze what you won't use right away.
- Eating in one place at home and at work.
- Never eat standing up.
- Make eating a singular activity; really enjoy and savor your food.
- Pause in the middle of your meal to check in with how you are feeling and how the food is tasting.
- Pay attention to your experience of eating. Make it pleasurable and sensual.
- Leave food on your plate if you are not hungry for it.
- Brush and floss your teeth when you feel like snacking and are not hungry.
- Share chores with your family; have them help put away leftovers.
- Plan ahead when it comes to eating out. Consider sharing an entree or having two appetizers.
- Bring Fido your leftovers!
- At parties, keep a glass of mineral water in your hands to prevent unnecessary eating.
- Eat breakfast every day.
- Move your body everyday.
- Relax yourself everyday.
- Take quiet time for yourself everyday.
- Treat yourself as you would your best friend.
- Exercise with someone to make it more fun.
- Establish an exercise routine that works with your lifestyle.
- Try exercising while watching TV or listening to music.
- Reward yourself often for your efforts towards a new and healthier lifestyle.

Speaking of your rewards, I prepared a fun "Rewards and Reinforcements" worksheet for you. You can find it in the Workbook section. The idea is to reward yourself for goals you reach, behaviors you change and challenges you meet. Using rewards is an excellent tool for success. Remember Sharon's piece of jewelry after her cruise?

Do you have any Tips For Success of your own? Add them here.

### *My Tips For Success*

_____

_____

_____

_____

_____

_____

_____

Part Four also includes a list entitled "Other Things to Do Instead of Eating". Use this list to remind yourself of the many activities and behaviors you can engage in when the emotional urge to eat strikes. Keep the list handy and refer to it often to get through some tight spots.

### Our Journey Together Draws to an End

We've come to the end of our fifteen weeks together. By completing this program you now have a better understanding of the relationship between your emotions and your eating. You have a set of skills and tools to carry you through any emotionally challenging time. You have the choice now whether to eat in response to your feelings or to choose another path. This has been an exciting time. You changed a lot. Your life changed a lot. If you continue on the path we started together, there is nothing you can't do!

# PART THREE:

## WHEN IT IS TIME TO SEE A PROFESSIONAL

Emotional eating, when its only symptom is overeating in response to stress, anxiety or other feelings, may be treated with a self-help method such as the one you are reading about here. More severe eating problems, such as anorexia, bulimia and binge eating disorders described in Part One require professional help.

### Getting Medical Attention
One way to determine if you need professional health is to take a look at the physical signs and symptoms of these disorders to see if you experience any of them. If you do, I urge you to seek professional medical help.

Here is a checklist of the physical symptoms you should be alert for.

#### Medical Signs and Symptoms Checklist
- Body Fluid Irregularities: potassium deficiencies; dehydration; low blood glucose
- Cardiovascular: slow pulse; heart irregularities; low blood pressure
- Dental: frequent cavities; teeth sensitivity; enamel erosion
- Edema: swelling; puffiness (usually around ankles and feet)
- Eyes: blurred vision; dark circles and puffiness
- Menstrual: Irregular periods; amennorhea; infertility
- Salivary Glands: swollen; painful; tender
- Skin: Patchy; dry; rashes; pimples; scaring on knuckles; fine lanugo hair
- Stomach: abdominal pain; bloating; fullness; irritable syndrome; constipation

### Getting Psychological Attention
There are psychological signs and symptoms that suggest the need for professional psychological help, even if you don't have a full-blown eating disorder. To assist you in determining if psychotherapy could help

you, I have prepared another checklist. If you find yourself suffering from any of these signs or symptoms, I encourage you to get psychological counseling. In the next section, I will show you how you go about finding competent care.

### Psychological Signs and Symptoms
* Binge eating
* Depression
* Diet pill use
* Dislike of your body
* Fasting
* Fear of eating in front of others
* Fear of gaining weight
* Feeling fat when you are an average weight
* Frequent dieting
* Guilt or shame after eating
* Irritability
* Isolation and withdrawal from friends and family
* Loss of control while eating
* Mood swings
* Overexercising
* Preference for strange foods or combinations of foods
* Preoccupation with weight and/or size
* Rapid eating
* Seeking an abnormally low body weight
* Sneak eating
* Strict dieting
* Suicidal thoughts
* Use of diuretics
* Use of laxative
* Vomiting
* Anxious feelings

◆ Panic attacks
◆ Unstable or unsatisfying relationships
◆ Fear of intimacy

## Choosing a Therapist

There are many different approaches to the treatment of eating disorders, and many different people and organizations offering services. Some involve in-patient care. Others are out-patient. The out-patient care can be through a hospital or a private practitioner. The most effective and long-lasting treatment plan is one that includes psychological counseling along with attention to medical and/or nutritional needs.

The best way to find a therapist is through a personal referral. Ask your doctors, clergy, family, and friends if they know anyone. If that fails to produce results, contact your local division of the American Psychological Association for help. You can peruse the yellow pages or display ads in your local papers. You can also contact a hospital in your area for assistance.

In choosing a therapist and the type of treatment you would like to have, consider asking the following questions:

◆ Do you treat anorexia nervosa, bulimia nervosa and/or other eating disorders?
◆ What kind of treatment do you provide?
◆ How long have you been treating eating disorders?
◆ What methods or combination of methods do you use?
◆ How successful are these methods?
◆ Are you licensed?
◆ What kind of license do you have?
◆ What are your credentials?
◆ Do you take insurance?

+ How will you evaluate me?
+ How much will this cost? (If their fees are too high, will they refer you to someone else?)
+ How long will the process take? When will I know I am finished with treatment?
+ Will I need a medical examination before we begin treatment?
+ What kind of medical information do you need?
+ What are the risks and benefits of choosing your type of treatment?
+ What are my alternatives?
+ Will you put me in the hospital?
+ Will I be on medication?
+ Will my family be involved?
+ Will my friends be involved?
+ Do you provide referrals if I need them?

In choosing a therapist, remember that rapport and confidence are just as important as credentials. Choose a therapist with whom you feel comfortable. Someone you feel you can trust to help you. Interview several therapists before settling on one. Ask for additional referrals if you need them.

### Finding a Support Group

In addition to finding a competent therapist to assist you in overcoming overeating, a support group can be a very valuable tool as well. Many therapists who treat eating issues have support groups because they are so effective in healing. If the therapist you have chosen does not have a support group, ask her if she knows of someone who does. Participate in both the personal therapy and the support group if you can. It is a highly effective way to beat this problem.

In a support groups you will hear how other people are overcoming overeating. You will learn new ways to cope with the issues in your life and you will experience a caring supportive environment to help you along the way.

You find a support group much the way you find a therapist, through referrals, yellow pages, newspaper ads, local hospitals, national associations, and so on. See the Resource section below for assistance.

If you cannot find a support group, you might consider starting your own. In Part Four, I give you a worksheet for starting your own group.

**Resources for Getting Help**
If you are still at a loss as to how to find a therapist, you can contact any of the resources listed here for additional help. I urge you to contact them anyway for additional information. Many of them send information free of charge so it is worth a quick phone call or postcard. I also left space for you to add the names, address and telephone numbers of any other resources that you learn of that I have not included.

- AED: Academy for Eating Disorders (703)556-9222; *www.acadeatdis.org;* an association of multi-disciplinary professionals
- AABA: American Anorexia/Bulimia Association (212)575-6200; *www.aabainc.org;* information and referrals
- American Anorexia and Bulimia Association (212-575-6200; 201-836-1800): provides support groups, referrals, and educational information
- American Dietetic Association (800-366-1655): referral service for nutritionists

- ANAD (National Association for Anorexia Nervosa and Associated Disorders) (847-831-3438): lists of therapists, hospitals, and sponsors groups
- Bulimia and Anorexia Self-help: (314) 567-4080
- Center for the Study of Anorexia and Bulimia: (212) 595-3449
- Council on Size and Weight Discrimination: (914) 679-1209
- EDAP: Eating Disorders Awareness and Prevention: (800) 931-2237; *www.edap.org;* information and referrals
- Gurze Books: (800) 756-7533: Catalogue of books and resources on eating disorders
- Harvard Eating Disorders Center: (617) 236-7766; *www.hedc.org;* research, information, newsletter
- Healing Connections, Inc.(212-585-3450): financial assistance available
- Healthy Weight Journal (701) 567-2646; newsletter
- IAEDP: International Association of Eating Disorders Professional: (800)800-8126; *www.iaedp.com;* referrals
- MEDA: Massachusetts Eating Disorders Association: (617)558-1881: referral network, local support groups
- National Anorexia Aid Society 614-436-1112
- NAAFA: National Association to Advance Fat Acceptance: (916)558-6880; *www.naafa.org;* information and newsletter
- National Health Information Center; (800) 994-9662 nationwide referrals and resource guides
- NEDSP: The National Eating Disorders Screening Program: (781)239-0071; kits of adults and teens
- Overeaters Anonymous (505-891-2664): free meetings in your area
- WINS: We Insist in Natural Shape (800)600-9467; *www.winsnews.org;* newsletters, videos
- *www.bulimia.com*: basic facts about eating disorders, national organizations and treatment facilities

**Treatment Facilities:**

- Binge Eating Program of the Western Psychiatric Institute and Clinic: (412) 624-2823; outpatient
- Canopy Cove: (800) 236-7524; *www.canopycove.com;* residential day treatment
- Center for Change: (888) 224-8250; *www.center for* change.com; inpatient
- Center for Discovery and Adolescent Change: (562) 425-7418; *www.centerfordiscovery.com;* residential program for teens
- Depaul Tulane Behavioral Health center: (800)548-4183; *www.depaultulane.com;* inpatient, partial and outpatient care
- Eating Disorder Center at Rogers Memorial Hospital; (800)767-4411; *www.rogershospital.org;* residential
- Eating Disorders Clinic of New York State Psychiatric Institute Columbia Presbyterian Medical Center: (212) 960-5739/5746; outpatient
- Eating Disorders Research Clinic of the University of Minnesota: (612) 627-4494; outpatient
- Eating Disorders Treatment Center at River Oaks Hospital: (800) 366-1740; *www.riveroakshospital.com*
- Hampstead Hospital: (800)600-5311; inpatient
- Institute for Living: (800)673-2411; inpatient and residential
- La Montagne: (636)931-3883; *www.lamontagne.org;* residential
- Laurel Hill: (781)396-1116; *www.laurelhill.com;* residential
- Mirasol: (888)520-1700; *www.mirasol.com;* alternative treatment facility
- Monet Nido: (310)457-9958; residential; also treats exercise addiction
- Montecatini: (760)436-8930; *www.montecatinieatingdisorder.com:* residential
- Nutrition Research Clinic of Baylor College of Medicine: (713)798-5757; outpatient

- Presbyterian Hospital of Dallas: (800)411-7081; *www.phscare.org;* inpatient
- Rader Programs: (800)841-1515; *www.raderprograms.com;* outpatient
- Remuda Ranch: (800)445-1900; *www.remuda-ranch.com;* residential
- Renfrew Center: (800-renfrew); *www.renfrew.org;* residential and outpatient
- Ridgeview Institute: (800)329-9775; *www.ridgeviewinstitute.com;* inpatient, residential, and outpatient
- River Centre Clinic: (419)885-8800; *www.river-centre.org;* outpatient
- Rosewood Ranch: (800)845-2211; *www.eatingdisorder.net;* residential
- Rutgers Eating Disorders Clinic: (908) 932-2292; outpatient;
- Shades of Hope: (800)588-HOPE: *www.shadesofhaope.com;* residential
- Sierra Tucson: (800)842-4487; *www.sierratucson.com:* residential
- Stanford University Department of Psychiatry: (415) 723-5868; inpatient and outpatient
- Wellspring: (203)266-8000; *www.wellspring.org;* residential
- Willough: (800)722-0100; *www.thewillough.com;* inpatient and outpatient
- Women's Recovery Center: (215) 664-5858; outpatient
- Yale Center for Eating and Weight Disorders: (203)432-4610: outpatient

If you are aware of other associations or resources that I have not included. List them here. This way you have all your information in one place.

## *Other Associations and Organizations*

_____

_____

_____

_____

_____

_____

_____

_____

_____

_____

# PART FOUR:

## THE DO YOU USE FOOD TO COPE WORKBOOK

## Food Awareness Inventory

The goal of the Food Awareness Inventory is to help you become aware of your current eating habits and triggers.

The inventory is very simple to use. For one week, itemize all the food you eat and beverages you drink. Using the chart below identify: the time you eat or drink; what you eat or drink; the amount consumed; and, any activity you were doing while eating or drinking.

At the end of the week you will review your inventory for patterns, trends, and other useful information about your eating habits. Remember, this is a tool for information not a weapon to beat yourself up with. If it starts to feel like an old diet habit of recording your food on a diary or if you start ridiculing yourself for your choices STOP! the exercise and do it some other time when you can be kinder to yourself.

## Food Awareness Inventory

| Day 1 | Time | Food/Beverage | Location | Activity |
|-------|------|---------------|----------|----------|
|       |      |               |          |          |
|       |      |               |          |          |
|       |      |               |          |          |
|       |      |               |          |          |
|       |      |               |          |          |
|       |      |               |          |          |
|       |      |               |          |          |
|       |      |               |          |          |
|       |      |               |          |          |
|       |      |               |          |          |
|       |      |               |          |          |
|       |      |               |          |          |
|       |      |               |          |          |
|       |      |               |          |          |
|       |      |               |          |          |
|       |      |               |          |          |
|       |      |               |          |          |
|       |      |               |          |          |

| Day 2 | Time | Food/Beverage | Location | Activity |
|-------|------|---------------|----------|----------|
|       |      |               |          |          |
|       |      |               |          |          |
|       |      |               |          |          |
|       |      |               |          |          |
|       |      |               |          |          |
|       |      |               |          |          |
|       |      |               |          |          |
|       |      |               |          |          |
|       |      |               |          |          |
|       |      |               |          |          |
|       |      |               |          |          |
|       |      |               |          |          |
|       |      |               |          |          |
|       |      |               |          |          |
|       |      |               |          |          |
|       |      |               |          |          |
|       |      |               |          |          |
|       |      |               |          |          |
|       |      |               |          |          |

| Day 3 | Time | Food/Beverage | Location | Activity |
|-------|------|---------------|----------|----------|
|       |      |               |          |          |
|       |      |               |          |          |
|       |      |               |          |          |
|       |      |               |          |          |
|       |      |               |          |          |
|       |      |               |          |          |
|       |      |               |          |          |
|       |      |               |          |          |
|       |      |               |          |          |
|       |      |               |          |          |
|       |      |               |          |          |
|       |      |               |          |          |
|       |      |               |          |          |
|       |      |               |          |          |
|       |      |               |          |          |
|       |      |               |          |          |
|       |      |               |          |          |
|       |      |               |          |          |
|       |      |               |          |          |

| Day 4 | Time | Food/Beverage | Location | Activity |
|-------|------|---------------|----------|----------|
|       |      |               |          |          |
|       |      |               |          |          |
|       |      |               |          |          |
|       |      |               |          |          |
|       |      |               |          |          |
|       |      |               |          |          |
|       |      |               |          |          |
|       |      |               |          |          |
|       |      |               |          |          |
|       |      |               |          |          |
|       |      |               |          |          |
|       |      |               |          |          |
|       |      |               |          |          |
|       |      |               |          |          |
|       |      |               |          |          |
|       |      |               |          |          |
|       |      |               |          |          |
|       |      |               |          |          |

| Day 5 | Time | Food/Beverage | Location | Activity |
|-------|------|---------------|----------|----------|
|       |      |               |          |          |
|       |      |               |          |          |
|       |      |               |          |          |
|       |      |               |          |          |
|       |      |               |          |          |
|       |      |               |          |          |
|       |      |               |          |          |
|       |      |               |          |          |
|       |      |               |          |          |
|       |      |               |          |          |
|       |      |               |          |          |
|       |      |               |          |          |
|       |      |               |          |          |
|       |      |               |          |          |
|       |      |               |          |          |
|       |      |               |          |          |
|       |      |               |          |          |
|       |      |               |          |          |
|       |      |               |          |          |

| Day 6 | Time | Food/Beverage | Location | Activity |
|-------|------|---------------|----------|----------|
|       |      |               |          |          |
|       |      |               |          |          |
|       |      |               |          |          |
|       |      |               |          |          |
|       |      |               |          |          |
|       |      |               |          |          |
|       |      |               |          |          |
|       |      |               |          |          |
|       |      |               |          |          |
|       |      |               |          |          |
|       |      |               |          |          |
|       |      |               |          |          |
|       |      |               |          |          |
|       |      |               |          |          |
|       |      |               |          |          |
|       |      |               |          |          |
|       |      |               |          |          |
|       |      |               |          |          |
|       |      |               |          |          |

| Day 7 | Time | Food/Beverage | Location | Activity |
|-------|------|---------------|----------|----------|
|       |      |               |          |          |
|       |      |               |          |          |
|       |      |               |          |          |
|       |      |               |          |          |
|       |      |               |          |          |
|       |      |               |          |          |
|       |      |               |          |          |
|       |      |               |          |          |
|       |      |               |          |          |
|       |      |               |          |          |
|       |      |               |          |          |
|       |      |               |          |          |
|       |      |               |          |          |
|       |      |               |          |          |
|       |      |               |          |          |
|       |      |               |          |          |
|       |      |               |          |          |
|       |      |               |          |          |
|       |      |               |          |          |

## Analysis: What I Learned About My Food Habits

*Overall:*

_____

_____

_____

_____

_____

_____

*Time:*

_____

_____

_____

_____

_____

_____

*Food/Beverages:*

_____

_____

_____

_____

_____

_____

*Location:*

_____

_____

_____
_____
_____
_____

*Activities:*

_____
_____
_____
_____
_____
_____

*Other:*

_____
_____
_____
_____
_____
_____

**Emotions Awareness Inventory**

Now you will learn more about how your emotions affect your eating habits. The goal of this inventory is to help you become aware of your moods when you eat. This inventory is also easy to use. It is just like the Food Awareness Inventory except that this week you will add a new category: "Feelings/Mood." And, again at the end of the week you will analyze your inventory for patterns, trends and insights.

Please remember that this inventory is for information only. If you find yourself judging yourself STOP! the exercise and continue some other time.

## *Emotions Awareness Inventory*

| Day 1 | Time | Food/Beverage | Location | Activity |
|---|---|---|---|---|
| | | | | |
| | | | | |
| | | | | |
| | | | | |
| | | | | |
| | | | | |
| | | | | |
| | | | | |
| | | | | |
| | | | | |
| | | | | |
| | | | | |
| | | | | |
| | | | | |
| | | | | |
| | | | | |
| | | | | |
| | | | | |

| Day 2 | Time | Food/Beverage | Location | Activity |
|-------|------|---------------|----------|----------|
|       |      |               |          |          |
|       |      |               |          |          |
|       |      |               |          |          |
|       |      |               |          |          |
|       |      |               |          |          |
|       |      |               |          |          |
|       |      |               |          |          |
|       |      |               |          |          |
|       |      |               |          |          |
|       |      |               |          |          |
|       |      |               |          |          |
|       |      |               |          |          |
|       |      |               |          |          |
|       |      |               |          |          |
|       |      |               |          |          |
|       |      |               |          |          |
|       |      |               |          |          |
|       |      |               |          |          |
|       |      |               |          |          |

| Day 3 | Time | Food/Beverage | Location | Activity |
|-------|------|---------------|----------|----------|
|       |      |               |          |          |
|       |      |               |          |          |
|       |      |               |          |          |
|       |      |               |          |          |
|       |      |               |          |          |
|       |      |               |          |          |
|       |      |               |          |          |
|       |      |               |          |          |
|       |      |               |          |          |
|       |      |               |          |          |
|       |      |               |          |          |
|       |      |               |          |          |
|       |      |               |          |          |
|       |      |               |          |          |
|       |      |               |          |          |
|       |      |               |          |          |
|       |      |               |          |          |
|       |      |               |          |          |

| Day 4 | Time | Food/Beverage | Location | Activity |
|-------|------|---------------|----------|----------|
|       |      |               |          |          |
|       |      |               |          |          |
|       |      |               |          |          |
|       |      |               |          |          |
|       |      |               |          |          |
|       |      |               |          |          |
|       |      |               |          |          |
|       |      |               |          |          |
|       |      |               |          |          |
|       |      |               |          |          |
|       |      |               |          |          |
|       |      |               |          |          |
|       |      |               |          |          |
|       |      |               |          |          |
|       |      |               |          |          |
|       |      |               |          |          |
|       |      |               |          |          |
|       |      |               |          |          |

| Day 5 | Time | Food/Beverage | Location | Activity |
|-------|------|---------------|----------|----------|
|       |      |               |          |          |
|       |      |               |          |          |
|       |      |               |          |          |
|       |      |               |          |          |
|       |      |               |          |          |
|       |      |               |          |          |
|       |      |               |          |          |
|       |      |               |          |          |
|       |      |               |          |          |
|       |      |               |          |          |
|       |      |               |          |          |
|       |      |               |          |          |
|       |      |               |          |          |
|       |      |               |          |          |
|       |      |               |          |          |
|       |      |               |          |          |
|       |      |               |          |          |
|       |      |               |          |          |

| Day 6 | Time | Food/Beverage | Location | Activity |
|-------|------|---------------|----------|----------|
|       |      |               |          |          |
|       |      |               |          |          |
|       |      |               |          |          |
|       |      |               |          |          |
|       |      |               |          |          |
|       |      |               |          |          |
|       |      |               |          |          |
|       |      |               |          |          |
|       |      |               |          |          |
|       |      |               |          |          |
|       |      |               |          |          |
|       |      |               |          |          |
|       |      |               |          |          |
|       |      |               |          |          |
|       |      |               |          |          |
|       |      |               |          |          |
|       |      |               |          |          |
|       |      |               |          |          |

| Day 7 | Time | Food/Beverage | Location | Activity |
|-------|------|---------------|----------|----------|
|       |      |               |          |          |
|       |      |               |          |          |
|       |      |               |          |          |
|       |      |               |          |          |
|       |      |               |          |          |
|       |      |               |          |          |
|       |      |               |          |          |
|       |      |               |          |          |
|       |      |               |          |          |
|       |      |               |          |          |
|       |      |               |          |          |
|       |      |               |          |          |
|       |      |               |          |          |
|       |      |               |          |          |
|       |      |               |          |          |
|       |      |               |          |          |
|       |      |               |          |          |
|       |      |               |          |          |
|       |      |               |          |          |

## Analysis: What I Learned About My Food and Moods

*Record Your Insights Here:*

_____
_____
_____
_____
_____
_____
_____
_____
_____
_____
_____
_____
_____

**My Hunger Inventory**

For this week you will record not only your food choices but also your hunger scale. Your hunger scale rates your hunger from 0 to 10. A 0 means that you are stuffed, like you just finished Thanksgiving dinner. A 10 means that you haven't eaten all day and if you don't get something into your stomach soon you'll faint. A 5 is being happily satisfied. You just ate a delicious meal and you are quite content. Using this scale of 0 to 10 keep track of your hunger this week.

| Day 1 | Time | Food/Beverage | Hunger Scale |
|-------|------|---------------|--------------|
|       |      |               |              |
|       |      |               |              |
|       |      |               |              |
|       |      |               |              |
|       |      |               |              |
|       |      |               |              |
|       |      |               |              |
|       |      |               |              |
|       |      |               |              |
|       |      |               |              |
|       |      |               |              |
|       |      |               |              |
|       |      |               |              |
|       |      |               |              |
|       |      |               |              |
|       |      |               |              |
|       |      |               |              |

| Day 2 | Time | Food/Beverage | Hunger Scale |
|-------|------|---------------|--------------|
|       |      |               |              |
|       |      |               |              |
|       |      |               |              |
|       |      |               |              |
|       |      |               |              |
|       |      |               |              |
|       |      |               |              |
|       |      |               |              |
|       |      |               |              |
|       |      |               |              |
|       |      |               |              |
|       |      |               |              |
|       |      |               |              |
|       |      |               |              |
|       |      |               |              |
|       |      |               |              |
|       |      |               |              |
|       |      |               |              |
|       |      |               |              |

| Day 3 | Time | Food/Beverage | Hunger Scale |
|---|---|---|---|
|  |  |  |  |
|  |  |  |  |
|  |  |  |  |
|  |  |  |  |
|  |  |  |  |
|  |  |  |  |
|  |  |  |  |
|  |  |  |  |
|  |  |  |  |
|  |  |  |  |
|  |  |  |  |
|  |  |  |  |
|  |  |  |  |
|  |  |  |  |
|  |  |  |  |
|  |  |  |  |
|  |  |  |  |
|  |  |  |  |

| Day 4 | Time | Food/Beverage | Hunger Scale |
|-------|------|---------------|--------------|
|       |      |               |              |
|       |      |               |              |
|       |      |               |              |
|       |      |               |              |
|       |      |               |              |
|       |      |               |              |
|       |      |               |              |
|       |      |               |              |
|       |      |               |              |
|       |      |               |              |
|       |      |               |              |
|       |      |               |              |
|       |      |               |              |
|       |      |               |              |
|       |      |               |              |
|       |      |               |              |
|       |      |               |              |
|       |      |               |              |

| Day 5 | Time | Food/Beverage | Hunger Scale |
|-------|------|---------------|--------------|
|       |      |               |              |
|       |      |               |              |
|       |      |               |              |
|       |      |               |              |
|       |      |               |              |
|       |      |               |              |
|       |      |               |              |
|       |      |               |              |
|       |      |               |              |
|       |      |               |              |
|       |      |               |              |
|       |      |               |              |
|       |      |               |              |
|       |      |               |              |
|       |      |               |              |
|       |      |               |              |
|       |      |               |              |
|       |      |               |              |

| Day 6 | Time | Food/Beverage | Hunger Scale |
|-------|------|---------------|--------------|
|       |      |               |              |
|       |      |               |              |
|       |      |               |              |
|       |      |               |              |
|       |      |               |              |
|       |      |               |              |
|       |      |               |              |
|       |      |               |              |
|       |      |               |              |
|       |      |               |              |
|       |      |               |              |
|       |      |               |              |
|       |      |               |              |
|       |      |               |              |
|       |      |               |              |
|       |      |               |              |
|       |      |               |              |
|       |      |               |              |
|       |      |               |              |

| Day 7 | Time | Food/Beverage | Hunger Scale |
|---|---|---|---|
| | | | |
| | | | |
| | | | |
| | | | |
| | | | |
| | | | |
| | | | |
| | | | |
| | | | |
| | | | |
| | | | |
| | | | |
| | | | |
| | | | |
| | | | |
| | | | |
| | | | |
| | | | |

## My Recovery Diary

| Day | Time | Food/Beverage | Location | Hunger | Emotion | Activity |
|-----|------|---------------|----------|--------|---------|----------|
| | | | | | | |
| | | | | | | |
| | | | | | | |
| | | | | | | |
| | | | | | | |
| | | | | | | |
| | | | | | | |
| | | | | | | |
| | | | | | | |
| | | | | | | |
| | | | | | | |
| | | | | | | |
| | | | | | | |
| | | | | | | |
| | | | | | | |
| | | | | | | |
| | | | | | | |
| | | | | | | |
| | | | | | | |
| | | | | | | |
| | | | | | | |
| | | | | | | |
| | | | | | | |
| | | | | | | |
| | | | | | | |
| | | | | | | |
| | | | | | | |
| | | | | | | |
| | | | | | | |
| | | | | | | |
| | | | | | | |
| | | | | | | |
| | | | | | | |
| | | | | | | |
| | | | | | | |
| | | | | | | |
| | | | | | | |
| | | | | | | |
| | | | | | | |
| | | | | | | |
| | | | | | | |

| Day | Time | Food/Beverage | Location | Hunger | Emotion | Activity |
|-----|------|---------------|----------|--------|---------|----------|
|     |      |               |          |        |         |          |
|     |      |               |          |        |         |          |
|     |      |               |          |        |         |          |
|     |      |               |          |        |         |          |
|     |      |               |          |        |         |          |
|     |      |               |          |        |         |          |
|     |      |               |          |        |         |          |
|     |      |               |          |        |         |          |
|     |      |               |          |        |         |          |
|     |      |               |          |        |         |          |
|     |      |               |          |        |         |          |
|     |      |               |          |        |         |          |
|     |      |               |          |        |         |          |
|     |      |               |          |        |         |          |
|     |      |               |          |        |         |          |
|     |      |               |          |        |         |          |
|     |      |               |          |        |         |          |
|     |      |               |          |        |         |          |
|     |      |               |          |        |         |          |
|     |      |               |          |        |         |          |
|     |      |               |          |        |         |          |
|     |      |               |          |        |         |          |
|     |      |               |          |        |         |          |
|     |      |               |          |        |         |          |
|     |      |               |          |        |         |          |
|     |      |               |          |        |         |          |
|     |      |               |          |        |         |          |
|     |      |               |          |        |         |          |
|     |      |               |          |        |         |          |
|     |      |               |          |        |         |          |
|     |      |               |          |        |         |          |
|     |      |               |          |        |         |          |
|     |      |               |          |        |         |          |
|     |      |               |          |        |         |          |
|     |      |               |          |        |         |          |
|     |      |               |          |        |         |          |
|     |      |               |          |        |         |          |
|     |      |               |          |        |         |          |
|     |      |               |          |        |         |          |
|     |      |               |          |        |         |          |

| Day | Time | Food/Beverage | Location | Hunger | Emotion | Activity |
|-----|------|---------------|----------|--------|---------|----------|
|  |  |  |  |  |  |  |
|  |  |  |  |  |  |  |
|  |  |  |  |  |  |  |
|  |  |  |  |  |  |  |
|  |  |  |  |  |  |  |
|  |  |  |  |  |  |  |
|  |  |  |  |  |  |  |
|  |  |  |  |  |  |  |
|  |  |  |  |  |  |  |
|  |  |  |  |  |  |  |
|  |  |  |  |  |  |  |
|  |  |  |  |  |  |  |
|  |  |  |  |  |  |  |
|  |  |  |  |  |  |  |
|  |  |  |  |  |  |  |
|  |  |  |  |  |  |  |
|  |  |  |  |  |  |  |
|  |  |  |  |  |  |  |
|  |  |  |  |  |  |  |
|  |  |  |  |  |  |  |
|  |  |  |  |  |  |  |
|  |  |  |  |  |  |  |
|  |  |  |  |  |  |  |
|  |  |  |  |  |  |  |
|  |  |  |  |  |  |  |
|  |  |  |  |  |  |  |
|  |  |  |  |  |  |  |
|  |  |  |  |  |  |  |
|  |  |  |  |  |  |  |
|  |  |  |  |  |  |  |
|  |  |  |  |  |  |  |
|  |  |  |  |  |  |  |
|  |  |  |  |  |  |  |
|  |  |  |  |  |  |  |
|  |  |  |  |  |  |  |
|  |  |  |  |  |  |  |
|  |  |  |  |  |  |  |
|  |  |  |  |  |  |  |
|  |  |  |  |  |  |  |
|  |  |  |  |  |  |  |
|  |  |  |  |  |  |  |

| Day | Time | Food/Beverage | Location | Hunger | Emotion | Activity |
|-----|------|---------------|----------|--------|---------|----------|
|     |      |               |          |        |         |          |
|     |      |               |          |        |         |          |
|     |      |               |          |        |         |          |
|     |      |               |          |        |         |          |
|     |      |               |          |        |         |          |
|     |      |               |          |        |         |          |
|     |      |               |          |        |         |          |
|     |      |               |          |        |         |          |
|     |      |               |          |        |         |          |
|     |      |               |          |        |         |          |
|     |      |               |          |        |         |          |
|     |      |               |          |        |         |          |
|     |      |               |          |        |         |          |
|     |      |               |          |        |         |          |
|     |      |               |          |        |         |          |
|     |      |               |          |        |         |          |
|     |      |               |          |        |         |          |
|     |      |               |          |        |         |          |
|     |      |               |          |        |         |          |
|     |      |               |          |        |         |          |
|     |      |               |          |        |         |          |
|     |      |               |          |        |         |          |
|     |      |               |          |        |         |          |
|     |      |               |          |        |         |          |
|     |      |               |          |        |         |          |
|     |      |               |          |        |         |          |
|     |      |               |          |        |         |          |
|     |      |               |          |        |         |          |
|     |      |               |          |        |         |          |
|     |      |               |          |        |         |          |
|     |      |               |          |        |         |          |
|     |      |               |          |        |         |          |
|     |      |               |          |        |         |          |
|     |      |               |          |        |         |          |
|     |      |               |          |        |         |          |
|     |      |               |          |        |         |          |
|     |      |               |          |        |         |          |
|     |      |               |          |        |         |          |
|     |      |               |          |        |         |          |
|     |      |               |          |        |         |          |

| Day | Time | Food/Beverage | Location | Hunger | Emotion | Activity |
|-----|------|---------------|----------|--------|---------|----------|
|  |  |  |  |  |  |  |
|  |  |  |  |  |  |  |
|  |  |  |  |  |  |  |
|  |  |  |  |  |  |  |
|  |  |  |  |  |  |  |
|  |  |  |  |  |  |  |
|  |  |  |  |  |  |  |
|  |  |  |  |  |  |  |
|  |  |  |  |  |  |  |
|  |  |  |  |  |  |  |
|  |  |  |  |  |  |  |
|  |  |  |  |  |  |  |
|  |  |  |  |  |  |  |
|  |  |  |  |  |  |  |
|  |  |  |  |  |  |  |
|  |  |  |  |  |  |  |
|  |  |  |  |  |  |  |
|  |  |  |  |  |  |  |
|  |  |  |  |  |  |  |
|  |  |  |  |  |  |  |
|  |  |  |  |  |  |  |
|  |  |  |  |  |  |  |
|  |  |  |  |  |  |  |
|  |  |  |  |  |  |  |
|  |  |  |  |  |  |  |
|  |  |  |  |  |  |  |
|  |  |  |  |  |  |  |
|  |  |  |  |  |  |  |
|  |  |  |  |  |  |  |
|  |  |  |  |  |  |  |
|  |  |  |  |  |  |  |
|  |  |  |  |  |  |  |
|  |  |  |  |  |  |  |
|  |  |  |  |  |  |  |
|  |  |  |  |  |  |  |
|  |  |  |  |  |  |  |
|  |  |  |  |  |  |  |
|  |  |  |  |  |  |  |
|  |  |  |  |  |  |  |
|  |  |  |  |  |  |  |
|  |  |  |  |  |  |  |

| Day | Time | Food/Beverage | Location | Hunger | Emotion | Activity |
|-----|------|---------------|----------|--------|---------|----------|
|     |      |               |          |        |         |          |
|     |      |               |          |        |         |          |
|     |      |               |          |        |         |          |
|     |      |               |          |        |         |          |
|     |      |               |          |        |         |          |
|     |      |               |          |        |         |          |
|     |      |               |          |        |         |          |
|     |      |               |          |        |         |          |
|     |      |               |          |        |         |          |
|     |      |               |          |        |         |          |
|     |      |               |          |        |         |          |
|     |      |               |          |        |         |          |
|     |      |               |          |        |         |          |
|     |      |               |          |        |         |          |
|     |      |               |          |        |         |          |
|     |      |               |          |        |         |          |
|     |      |               |          |        |         |          |
|     |      |               |          |        |         |          |
|     |      |               |          |        |         |          |
|     |      |               |          |        |         |          |
|     |      |               |          |        |         |          |
|     |      |               |          |        |         |          |
|     |      |               |          |        |         |          |
|     |      |               |          |        |         |          |
|     |      |               |          |        |         |          |
|     |      |               |          |        |         |          |
|     |      |               |          |        |         |          |
|     |      |               |          |        |         |          |
|     |      |               |          |        |         |          |
|     |      |               |          |        |         |          |
|     |      |               |          |        |         |          |
|     |      |               |          |        |         |          |
|     |      |               |          |        |         |          |
|     |      |               |          |        |         |          |
|     |      |               |          |        |         |          |
|     |      |               |          |        |         |          |
|     |      |               |          |        |         |          |
|     |      |               |          |        |         |          |
|     |      |               |          |        |         |          |
|     |      |               |          |        |         |          |
|     |      |               |          |        |         |          |
|     |      |               |          |        |         |          |
|     |      |               |          |        |         |          |
|     |      |               |          |        |         |          |

| Day | Time | Food/Beverage | Location | Hunger | Emotion | Activity |
|-----|------|---------------|----------|--------|---------|----------|
|     |      |               |          |        |         |          |
|     |      |               |          |        |         |          |
|     |      |               |          |        |         |          |
|     |      |               |          |        |         |          |
|     |      |               |          |        |         |          |
|     |      |               |          |        |         |          |
|     |      |               |          |        |         |          |
|     |      |               |          |        |         |          |
|     |      |               |          |        |         |          |
|     |      |               |          |        |         |          |
|     |      |               |          |        |         |          |
|     |      |               |          |        |         |          |
|     |      |               |          |        |         |          |
|     |      |               |          |        |         |          |
|     |      |               |          |        |         |          |
|     |      |               |          |        |         |          |
|     |      |               |          |        |         |          |
|     |      |               |          |        |         |          |
|     |      |               |          |        |         |          |
|     |      |               |          |        |         |          |
|     |      |               |          |        |         |          |
|     |      |               |          |        |         |          |
|     |      |               |          |        |         |          |
|     |      |               |          |        |         |          |
|     |      |               |          |        |         |          |
|     |      |               |          |        |         |          |
|     |      |               |          |        |         |          |
|     |      |               |          |        |         |          |
|     |      |               |          |        |         |          |
|     |      |               |          |        |         |          |
|     |      |               |          |        |         |          |
|     |      |               |          |        |         |          |
|     |      |               |          |        |         |          |
|     |      |               |          |        |         |          |
|     |      |               |          |        |         |          |
|     |      |               |          |        |         |          |
|     |      |               |          |        |         |          |
|     |      |               |          |        |         |          |
|     |      |               |          |        |         |          |
|     |      |               |          |        |         |          |

| Day | Time | Food/Beverage | Location | Hunger | Emotion | Activity |
|-----|------|---------------|----------|--------|---------|----------|
|     |      |               |          |        |         |          |
|     |      |               |          |        |         |          |
|     |      |               |          |        |         |          |
|     |      |               |          |        |         |          |
|     |      |               |          |        |         |          |
|     |      |               |          |        |         |          |
|     |      |               |          |        |         |          |
|     |      |               |          |        |         |          |
|     |      |               |          |        |         |          |
|     |      |               |          |        |         |          |
|     |      |               |          |        |         |          |
|     |      |               |          |        |         |          |
|     |      |               |          |        |         |          |
|     |      |               |          |        |         |          |
|     |      |               |          |        |         |          |
|     |      |               |          |        |         |          |
|     |      |               |          |        |         |          |
|     |      |               |          |        |         |          |
|     |      |               |          |        |         |          |
|     |      |               |          |        |         |          |
|     |      |               |          |        |         |          |
|     |      |               |          |        |         |          |
|     |      |               |          |        |         |          |
|     |      |               |          |        |         |          |
|     |      |               |          |        |         |          |
|     |      |               |          |        |         |          |
|     |      |               |          |        |         |          |
|     |      |               |          |        |         |          |
|     |      |               |          |        |         |          |
|     |      |               |          |        |         |          |
|     |      |               |          |        |         |          |
|     |      |               |          |        |         |          |
|     |      |               |          |        |         |          |
|     |      |               |          |        |         |          |
|     |      |               |          |        |         |          |
|     |      |               |          |        |         |          |
|     |      |               |          |        |         |          |
|     |      |               |          |        |         |          |
|     |      |               |          |        |         |          |
|     |      |               |          |        |         |          |
|     |      |               |          |        |         |          |
|     |      |               |          |        |         |          |

| Day | Time | Food/Beverage | Location | Hunger | Emotion | Activity |
|-----|------|---------------|----------|--------|---------|----------|
|     |      |               |          |        |         |          |
|     |      |               |          |        |         |          |
|     |      |               |          |        |         |          |
|     |      |               |          |        |         |          |
|     |      |               |          |        |         |          |
|     |      |               |          |        |         |          |
|     |      |               |          |        |         |          |
|     |      |               |          |        |         |          |
|     |      |               |          |        |         |          |
|     |      |               |          |        |         |          |
|     |      |               |          |        |         |          |
|     |      |               |          |        |         |          |
|     |      |               |          |        |         |          |
|     |      |               |          |        |         |          |
|     |      |               |          |        |         |          |
|     |      |               |          |        |         |          |
|     |      |               |          |        |         |          |
|     |      |               |          |        |         |          |
|     |      |               |          |        |         |          |
|     |      |               |          |        |         |          |
|     |      |               |          |        |         |          |
|     |      |               |          |        |         |          |
|     |      |               |          |        |         |          |
|     |      |               |          |        |         |          |
|     |      |               |          |        |         |          |
|     |      |               |          |        |         |          |
|     |      |               |          |        |         |          |
|     |      |               |          |        |         |          |
|     |      |               |          |        |         |          |
|     |      |               |          |        |         |          |
|     |      |               |          |        |         |          |
|     |      |               |          |        |         |          |
|     |      |               |          |        |         |          |
|     |      |               |          |        |         |          |
|     |      |               |          |        |         |          |
|     |      |               |          |        |         |          |
|     |      |               |          |        |         |          |
|     |      |               |          |        |         |          |
|     |      |               |          |        |         |          |
|     |      |               |          |        |         |          |
|     |      |               |          |        |         |          |

| Day | Time | Food/Beverage | Location | Hunger | Emotion | Activity |
|-----|------|---------------|----------|--------|---------|----------|
|     |      |               |          |        |         |          |
|     |      |               |          |        |         |          |
|     |      |               |          |        |         |          |
|     |      |               |          |        |         |          |
|     |      |               |          |        |         |          |
|     |      |               |          |        |         |          |
|     |      |               |          |        |         |          |
|     |      |               |          |        |         |          |
|     |      |               |          |        |         |          |
|     |      |               |          |        |         |          |
|     |      |               |          |        |         |          |
|     |      |               |          |        |         |          |
|     |      |               |          |        |         |          |
|     |      |               |          |        |         |          |
|     |      |               |          |        |         |          |
|     |      |               |          |        |         |          |
|     |      |               |          |        |         |          |
|     |      |               |          |        |         |          |
|     |      |               |          |        |         |          |
|     |      |               |          |        |         |          |
|     |      |               |          |        |         |          |
|     |      |               |          |        |         |          |
|     |      |               |          |        |         |          |
|     |      |               |          |        |         |          |
|     |      |               |          |        |         |          |
|     |      |               |          |        |         |          |
|     |      |               |          |        |         |          |
|     |      |               |          |        |         |          |
|     |      |               |          |        |         |          |
|     |      |               |          |        |         |          |
|     |      |               |          |        |         |          |
|     |      |               |          |        |         |          |
|     |      |               |          |        |         |          |
|     |      |               |          |        |         |          |
|     |      |               |          |        |         |          |
|     |      |               |          |        |         |          |
|     |      |               |          |        |         |          |
|     |      |               |          |        |         |          |
|     |      |               |          |        |         |          |
|     |      |               |          |        |         |          |
|     |      |               |          |        |         |          |

| Day | Time | Food/Beverage | Location | Hunger | Emotion | Activity |
|-----|------|---------------|----------|--------|---------|----------|
|     |      |               |          |        |         |          |
|     |      |               |          |        |         |          |
|     |      |               |          |        |         |          |
|     |      |               |          |        |         |          |
|     |      |               |          |        |         |          |
|     |      |               |          |        |         |          |
|     |      |               |          |        |         |          |
|     |      |               |          |        |         |          |
|     |      |               |          |        |         |          |
|     |      |               |          |        |         |          |
|     |      |               |          |        |         |          |
|     |      |               |          |        |         |          |
|     |      |               |          |        |         |          |
|     |      |               |          |        |         |          |
|     |      |               |          |        |         |          |
|     |      |               |          |        |         |          |
|     |      |               |          |        |         |          |
|     |      |               |          |        |         |          |
|     |      |               |          |        |         |          |
|     |      |               |          |        |         |          |
|     |      |               |          |        |         |          |
|     |      |               |          |        |         |          |
|     |      |               |          |        |         |          |
|     |      |               |          |        |         |          |
|     |      |               |          |        |         |          |
|     |      |               |          |        |         |          |
|     |      |               |          |        |         |          |
|     |      |               |          |        |         |          |
|     |      |               |          |        |         |          |
|     |      |               |          |        |         |          |
|     |      |               |          |        |         |          |
|     |      |               |          |        |         |          |
|     |      |               |          |        |         |          |
|     |      |               |          |        |         |          |
|     |      |               |          |        |         |          |
|     |      |               |          |        |         |          |
|     |      |               |          |        |         |          |
|     |      |               |          |        |         |          |
|     |      |               |          |        |         |          |
|     |      |               |          |        |         |          |
|     |      |               |          |        |         |          |
|     |      |               |          |        |         |          |

| Day | Time | Food/Beverage | Location | Hunger | Emotion | Activity |
|-----|------|---------------|----------|--------|---------|----------|
|     |      |               |          |        |         |          |
|     |      |               |          |        |         |          |
|     |      |               |          |        |         |          |
|     |      |               |          |        |         |          |
|     |      |               |          |        |         |          |
|     |      |               |          |        |         |          |
|     |      |               |          |        |         |          |
|     |      |               |          |        |         |          |
|     |      |               |          |        |         |          |
|     |      |               |          |        |         |          |
|     |      |               |          |        |         |          |
|     |      |               |          |        |         |          |
|     |      |               |          |        |         |          |
|     |      |               |          |        |         |          |
|     |      |               |          |        |         |          |
|     |      |               |          |        |         |          |
|     |      |               |          |        |         |          |
|     |      |               |          |        |         |          |
|     |      |               |          |        |         |          |
|     |      |               |          |        |         |          |
|     |      |               |          |        |         |          |
|     |      |               |          |        |         |          |
|     |      |               |          |        |         |          |
|     |      |               |          |        |         |          |
|     |      |               |          |        |         |          |
|     |      |               |          |        |         |          |
|     |      |               |          |        |         |          |
|     |      |               |          |        |         |          |
|     |      |               |          |        |         |          |
|     |      |               |          |        |         |          |
|     |      |               |          |        |         |          |
|     |      |               |          |        |         |          |
|     |      |               |          |        |         |          |
|     |      |               |          |        |         |          |
|     |      |               |          |        |         |          |
|     |      |               |          |        |         |          |
|     |      |               |          |        |         |          |
|     |      |               |          |        |         |          |
|     |      |               |          |        |         |          |
|     |      |               |          |        |         |          |
|     |      |               |          |        |         |          |
|     |      |               |          |        |         |          |
|     |      |               |          |        |         |          |

| Day | Time | Food/Beverage | Location | Hunger | Emotion | Activity |
|-----|------|---------------|----------|--------|---------|----------|
|     |      |               |          |        |         |          |
|     |      |               |          |        |         |          |
|     |      |               |          |        |         |          |
|     |      |               |          |        |         |          |
|     |      |               |          |        |         |          |
|     |      |               |          |        |         |          |
|     |      |               |          |        |         |          |
|     |      |               |          |        |         |          |
|     |      |               |          |        |         |          |
|     |      |               |          |        |         |          |
|     |      |               |          |        |         |          |
|     |      |               |          |        |         |          |
|     |      |               |          |        |         |          |
|     |      |               |          |        |         |          |
|     |      |               |          |        |         |          |
|     |      |               |          |        |         |          |
|     |      |               |          |        |         |          |
|     |      |               |          |        |         |          |
|     |      |               |          |        |         |          |
|     |      |               |          |        |         |          |
|     |      |               |          |        |         |          |
|     |      |               |          |        |         |          |
|     |      |               |          |        |         |          |
|     |      |               |          |        |         |          |
|     |      |               |          |        |         |          |
|     |      |               |          |        |         |          |
|     |      |               |          |        |         |          |
|     |      |               |          |        |         |          |
|     |      |               |          |        |         |          |
|     |      |               |          |        |         |          |
|     |      |               |          |        |         |          |
|     |      |               |          |        |         |          |
|     |      |               |          |        |         |          |
|     |      |               |          |        |         |          |
|     |      |               |          |        |         |          |
|     |      |               |          |        |         |          |
|     |      |               |          |        |         |          |
|     |      |               |          |        |         |          |
|     |      |               |          |        |         |          |
|     |      |               |          |        |         |          |
|     |      |               |          |        |         |          |
|     |      |               |          |        |         |          |
|     |      |               |          |        |         |          |
|     |      |               |          |        |         |          |
|     |      |               |          |        |         |          |
|     |      |               |          |        |         |          |

| Day | Time | Food/Beverage | Location | Hunger | Emotion | Activity |
|---|---|---|---|---|---|---|
| | | | | | | |
| | | | | | | |
| | | | | | | |
| | | | | | | |
| | | | | | | |
| | | | | | | |
| | | | | | | |
| | | | | | | |
| | | | | | | |
| | | | | | | |
| | | | | | | |
| | | | | | | |
| | | | | | | |
| | | | | | | |
| | | | | | | |
| | | | | | | |
| | | | | | | |
| | | | | | | |
| | | | | | | |
| | | | | | | |
| | | | | | | |
| | | | | | | |
| | | | | | | |
| | | | | | | |
| | | | | | | |
| | | | | | | |
| | | | | | | |
| | | | | | | |
| | | | | | | |
| | | | | | | |
| | | | | | | |
| | | | | | | |
| | | | | | | |
| | | | | | | |
| | | | | | | |
| | | | | | | |
| | | | | | | |
| | | | | | | |
| | | | | | | |
| | | | | | | |

| Day | Time | Food/Beverage | Location | Hunger | Emotion | Activity |
|-----|------|---------------|----------|--------|---------|----------|
|     |      |               |          |        |         |          |
|     |      |               |          |        |         |          |
|     |      |               |          |        |         |          |
|     |      |               |          |        |         |          |
|     |      |               |          |        |         |          |
|     |      |               |          |        |         |          |
|     |      |               |          |        |         |          |
|     |      |               |          |        |         |          |
|     |      |               |          |        |         |          |
|     |      |               |          |        |         |          |
|     |      |               |          |        |         |          |
|     |      |               |          |        |         |          |
|     |      |               |          |        |         |          |
|     |      |               |          |        |         |          |
|     |      |               |          |        |         |          |
|     |      |               |          |        |         |          |
|     |      |               |          |        |         |          |
|     |      |               |          |        |         |          |
|     |      |               |          |        |         |          |
|     |      |               |          |        |         |          |
|     |      |               |          |        |         |          |
|     |      |               |          |        |         |          |
|     |      |               |          |        |         |          |
|     |      |               |          |        |         |          |
|     |      |               |          |        |         |          |
|     |      |               |          |        |         |          |
|     |      |               |          |        |         |          |
|     |      |               |          |        |         |          |
|     |      |               |          |        |         |          |
|     |      |               |          |        |         |          |
|     |      |               |          |        |         |          |
|     |      |               |          |        |         |          |
|     |      |               |          |        |         |          |
|     |      |               |          |        |         |          |
|     |      |               |          |        |         |          |
|     |      |               |          |        |         |          |

| Day | Time | Food/Beverage | Location | Hunger | Emotion | Activity |
|-----|------|---------------|----------|--------|---------|----------|
|     |      |               |          |        |         |          |
|     |      |               |          |        |         |          |
|     |      |               |          |        |         |          |
|     |      |               |          |        |         |          |
|     |      |               |          |        |         |          |
|     |      |               |          |        |         |          |
|     |      |               |          |        |         |          |
|     |      |               |          |        |         |          |
|     |      |               |          |        |         |          |
|     |      |               |          |        |         |          |
|     |      |               |          |        |         |          |
|     |      |               |          |        |         |          |
|     |      |               |          |        |         |          |
|     |      |               |          |        |         |          |
|     |      |               |          |        |         |          |
|     |      |               |          |        |         |          |
|     |      |               |          |        |         |          |
|     |      |               |          |        |         |          |
|     |      |               |          |        |         |          |
|     |      |               |          |        |         |          |
|     |      |               |          |        |         |          |
|     |      |               |          |        |         |          |
|     |      |               |          |        |         |          |
|     |      |               |          |        |         |          |
|     |      |               |          |        |         |          |
|     |      |               |          |        |         |          |
|     |      |               |          |        |         |          |
|     |      |               |          |        |         |          |
|     |      |               |          |        |         |          |
|     |      |               |          |        |         |          |
|     |      |               |          |        |         |          |
|     |      |               |          |        |         |          |
|     |      |               |          |        |         |          |
|     |      |               |          |        |         |          |
|     |      |               |          |        |         |          |
|     |      |               |          |        |         |          |
|     |      |               |          |        |         |          |
|     |      |               |          |        |         |          |
|     |      |               |          |        |         |          |
|     |      |               |          |        |         |          |

| Day | Time | Food/Beverage | Location | Hunger | Emotion | Activity |
|-----|------|---------------|----------|--------|---------|----------|
|     |      |               |          |        |         |          |
|     |      |               |          |        |         |          |
|     |      |               |          |        |         |          |
|     |      |               |          |        |         |          |
|     |      |               |          |        |         |          |
|     |      |               |          |        |         |          |
|     |      |               |          |        |         |          |
|     |      |               |          |        |         |          |
|     |      |               |          |        |         |          |
|     |      |               |          |        |         |          |
|     |      |               |          |        |         |          |
|     |      |               |          |        |         |          |
|     |      |               |          |        |         |          |
|     |      |               |          |        |         |          |
|     |      |               |          |        |         |          |
|     |      |               |          |        |         |          |
|     |      |               |          |        |         |          |
|     |      |               |          |        |         |          |
|     |      |               |          |        |         |          |
|     |      |               |          |        |         |          |
|     |      |               |          |        |         |          |
|     |      |               |          |        |         |          |
|     |      |               |          |        |         |          |
|     |      |               |          |        |         |          |
|     |      |               |          |        |         |          |
|     |      |               |          |        |         |          |
|     |      |               |          |        |         |          |
|     |      |               |          |        |         |          |
|     |      |               |          |        |         |          |
|     |      |               |          |        |         |          |
|     |      |               |          |        |         |          |
|     |      |               |          |        |         |          |
|     |      |               |          |        |         |          |
|     |      |               |          |        |         |          |
|     |      |               |          |        |         |          |
|     |      |               |          |        |         |          |
|     |      |               |          |        |         |          |
|     |      |               |          |        |         |          |
|     |      |               |          |        |         |          |
|     |      |               |          |        |         |          |

## Plan of Action Worksheet

A Plan of Action carefully created and faithfully implemented can go a long away to preventing lapses and relapses. Use this worksheet to design your own course of action for any obstacles you may encounter on your road to overcoming emotional overeating.

**Anticipated Obstacle:**

_____

_____

_____

_____

_____

**Steps to Take to Handle it:**

_____

_____

_____

_____

_____

**Time Frame for Action:**

_____

_____

_____

_____

_____

## My "Other Things To Do Instead of Eating" List

Use this list to remind yourself of activities and behaviors you can enjoy when the urge to eat emotionally strikes you. I started the list with some ideas of my own. You fill in the rest. Personalize it so it has special value to you.

1. Take a bath.

2. Take a walk.

3. Write a letter.

4. _____

5. _____

6. _____

7. _____

8. _____

9. _____

10. _____

11. _____

12. _____

13. _____

14. _____

15. _____

16. _____

17. _____

18. _____

## Anger Letter

Dear _____,

_____

_____

_____

_____

_____

_____

_____

_____

_____

_____

_____

_____

_____

_____

_____

_____

_____

_____

_____

_____

_____

_____

_____

_____

_____

_____

Signed,

_____

## Love Myself Letter

Dear Me,

_____

_____

_____

_____

_____

_____

_____

_____

_____

_____

_____

_____

_____

_____

_____

_____

_____

_____

_____

_____

_____

_____

_____

_____

_____

Love,

Me

# My Journal

## Rewards and Reinforcements

Give yourself 1 point each time you meet a goal, change a behavior, or do something challenging. For example, give yourself a point each time you eat when you hungry, stop when you are full, do something else instead of eat, take a walk, or assert yourself. At the end of each week reward yourself in 5 point increments.

For example :
- 5 points: Take a bubble bath
- 10 points: Treat yourself to a new book
- 15 points: Get a manicure
- 20 points: Get a pedicure
- 100 points: Go to Palm Springs for the weekend

Now fill in your "Rewards and Reinforcements".

### *My Rewards and Reinforcements*

5 points : _____
10 points: _____
15 points: _____
20 points: _____
25 points: _____
30 points: _____
35 points: _____
40 points: _____
45 points: _____
50 points: _____
55 points: _____
60 points: _____
65 points: _____
70 points: _____
75 points: _____
80 points: _____
85 points: _____

90 points: _____
95 points: _____
100 points: _____

## Rewards Chart

| Week | Rewards | Week | Rewards |
|------|---------|------|---------|
|      |         |      |         |
|      |         |      |         |
|      |         |      |         |
|      |         |      |         |
|      |         |      |         |
|      |         |      |         |
|      |         |      |         |
|      |         |      |         |
|      |         |      |         |
|      |         |      |         |
|      |         |      |         |
|      |         |      |         |

Or, you can reward yourself with money at the end of each week. You set the goals and the amounts. Then put the money into a special envelop each week. At the end of the year....splurge!

## Financial Rewards Chart

| Week | Amount | Week | Amount |
|------|--------|------|--------|
|      |        |      |        |
|      |        |      |        |
|      |        |      |        |
|      |        |      |        |
|      |        |      |        |
|      |        |      |        |
|      |        |      |        |
|      |        |      |        |
|      |        |      |        |
|      |        |      |        |
|      |        |      |        |
|      |        |      |        |
|      |        |      |        |

## Goal Setting Worksheet
### 5 Year Goals

Work/Career: _____

Financial: _____

Love/Relationships: _____

Education: _____

Lifestyle: _____

Travel: _____

Leisure: _____

Personal Growth: _____

Health: _____

Other: _____

One Year Goals

_____
_____
_____
_____
_____
_____

6 Month Goals

_____
_____
_____
_____
_____
_____

3 Month Goals

_____
_____
_____
_____
_____
_____

1 Month Goals

_____
_____
_____
_____
_____
_____

## 1 Week Goals

_____
_____
_____
_____
_____
_____
_____

## Daily Goals

_____
_____
_____
_____
_____
_____

Notes/Comments:

_____
_____
_____
_____
_____
_____
_____

**Forming Your Own Support Group**

Here are the 10 easy steps to forming your own Support Group:

- Talk to friends, colleagues, and relatives you know who have problems with food and find out if they would be interested in forming a support group to overcome these problems.
- Put an ad in your local paper to recruit more members. Try to keep your number of members between 6 and 10.
- Decide on a day, time, and place to meet.
- Distribute a copy of Do You Use Food to Cope? to each member.
- Assign a certain number of pages to read for each meeting.
- Read the assigned pages and the exercises contained within them.
- Use the assignments and exercises as a starting point for your meeting.
- Allow each member her turn to participate.
- Rotate leaders/ facilitators weekly.
- Most important, allow free range of emotions and efforts so the members feel safe to share their experiences, deepest concerns, and feelings.

**Photojournalism:**
**Instructions for Creating Image Pages**

Get a large piece of poster board. Using old photographs, magazine clippings, or your own drawings, paste pictures, word, and images that reflect the self and the life you would like to create. Include everything you would like to have, be, or achieve. For example:

- The car you would like to drive.
- The clothes you would like to wear.
- The house you would like to live in.
- The job you would like to get.

- The feelings you would like to experience.
- The relationships you would like to see yourself in.

Feel free to use separate pages for each image you would like to create or you can make one big collage.

## Refrigerator Tear Out

(Tear out and place on refrigerator or pantry door)

# *WHAT'S GOING ON?*

# *WHAT AM I FEELING?*

# *WHAT DO I REALLY NEED?*

# *HOW CAN I MEET MY NEEDS WITHOUT OVEREATING?*

## Other Strategies

1.  Tape record feelings.

2.  Write a letter (which you don't mail or deliver) to someone you need to address.

3.  _____

4.  _____

5.  _____

6.  _____

7.  _____

8.  _____

9.  _____

10. _____

# ABOUT THE AUTHOR

Dr. Sheila H. Forman is both a licensed psychologist and attorney. She maintains a private clinical psychology practice in Santa Monica California where she specializes in the use of group and individual psychotherapy for the treatment of anxiety, depression and eating disorders. She is a member of many professional associations including the International Association of Eating Disorder Professionals and the Anorexia Nervosa and Related Disorders Association. She teaches classes on the diagnosis and treatment of eating disorders to mental health professionals and is the author of *Self-fullness: the Art of Loving and Caring for Your "Self"*.

*Self-help/Psychology* $15.95

*Are You*:

- Turning to food when you feel tired, stressed, sad, overwhelmed or angry?
- Tried of struggling with your weight?
- Unhappy with your body and physical appearance?
- Frustrated with repeated diet failures?
- Consumed by cravings for high-fat and high-sugar foods when you are under stress?
- Ready to address the issues underlying your overeating?
- Willing to take the next 15 weeks to change your life?

Then, **DO YOU USE FOOD TO COPE? A Comprehensive 15-Week Program for Overcoming Emotional Overeating** is for you!

Drawing upon years of research and clinical experience, Dr. Sheila H. Forman, clinical psychologist and eating disorder specialist, has created a thorough and easy to follow 15-week program to help you let go of emotional eating. Week by week, Dr. Forman takes you through the steps necessary to understand the relationship between your emotions and food. By the end of the 15 weeks you will have a plan for dealing with your emotional life without turning to food as a coping mechanism.

*Not A Diet But A New Way of Life!*

www.ingramcontent.com/pod-product-compliance
Lightning Source LLC
Chambersburg PA
CBHW061356280526
45784CB00001B/275